The 5-Stage Program for Permanent Weight Loss

# the complete
# Beck
# diet for
# life

Featuring
*The Think Thin
Eating Plan*

*New York Times* Bestselling Author
## Judith S. Beck, Ph.D.

The 5-Stage Program for Permanent Weight Loss

the complete

# Beck
# diet for
# life

Featuring
*The Think Thin
Eating Plan*

*New York Times* Bestselling Author
## Judith S. Beck, Ph.D.

Beck Institute for Cognitive Therapy and Research
Clinical Associate Professor of Psychology in Psychiatry
University of Pennsylvania

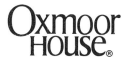

Oxmoor
House®

Published by Oxmoor House, Inc.
Book Division of Southern Progress Corporation
P.O. Box 2262, Birmingham, Alabama 35201-2262

ISBN-13: 978-0-8487-3274-5
ISBN-10: 0-8487-3274-X
Library of Congress Control Number: 2008934130
Printed in the United States of America
First Printing 2008

Be sure to check with your health-care provider before making any changes in your diet or exercise routine.

Editorial and Production Support: L. Amanda Owens, Melissa Jones Clark, Vanessa Rusch Thomas, Allison Long Lowery, Laura Lockhart, Greg A. Amason

Cover Image: Siri Stafford/Getty Images
Cover Design: Joline Rivera

To order additional publications, call 1-800-765-6400.

For more books to enrich your life, **visit oxmoorhouse.com**

*To my daughter, Deborah Beck Busis*

# Contents

# Acknowledgments

What a great pleasure it has been collaborating with my daughter Deborah Beck Busis in writing this book. Debbie and I had countless discussions, virtually every day, about our respective dieters: their sabotaging thoughts and habits; their struggles and successes; the techniques we were developing to help them overcome psychological and practical obstacles—and about how best to present this material in a reader-friendly way so dieters could lose weight on their own. So great thanks to Debbie for her endless supply of creative and valuable ideas, for co-leading workshops on the topic, and for her polished writing and editorial skills.

Many thanks to my husband, Richard Busis, whose unending support (and editing) made this a better book; to Alisa Bowman, who helped to organize the material; to Tracy Gensler, R.D., who helped to refine the eating plans and develop the recipes; to my friends who tested the recipes; and to Beth Grossman and Meryl Moss who publicized the book. As always, I'm grateful to my wonderful Oxmoor House team: Amanda Owens, Melissa Clark, Vanessa Rusch Thomas, Sydney Webber, Jim Childs, and Brian Carnahan. A special thanks to Stephanie Tade, agent extraordinaire, whose assistance has been so essential, every step of the way.

I would also like to thank my excellent staff at the Beck Institute for Cognitive Therapy and Research, with special thanks to Naomi Dank, Ph.D., who has always given 150 percent so I could devote time to writing. Thanks, too, to my mother, Phyllis Beck, for encouraging me in every possible way and to my father, Aaron Beck, with whom I have had the pleasure and honor of discussing, since a young age, the field he created: Cognitive Therapy.

Finally, I would like to thank the thousands of dieters, diet coaches, and health and mental-health professionals who have e-mailed me, or whose blogs and Internet discussion-group postings Debbie and I have read. Their messages have enriched our thinking and influenced many aspects of this book.

# Introduction

I am glad you have found your way to this book. I think you will find it very different from other approaches to weight loss. Most programs just tell you what to eat and what not to eat. But as research bears out, that is rarely enough. The difficult part of dieting is actually *sticking* to a diet. *The Complete Beck Diet for Life* not only provides you with a highly nutritious, enjoyable diet (which includes your favorite foods), but also teaches you how to motivate yourself to follow it—day after day after day.

It's not surprising to me that you probably have had difficulty either losing excess weight or keeping it off. The problem is that no one ever taught you *how* to diet. Most people can lose some weight by biting the bullet and restricting their eating for a period of time, but almost everyone gains it back. They just don't know what to do when they are feeling upset, stressed, or tired; when their lives get too busy; when hunger and cravings intensify; when they eat out; when people push food on them; and when it just doesn't seem worth it anymore. Through a step-by-step program, *The Complete Beck Diet for Life* addresses all of these problems and more, teaching you the skills you need to achieve permanent weight loss.

My first books on dieting, *The Beck Diet Solution* and *The Beck Diet Solution Weight Loss Workbook,* struck a chord with dieters. To date, they have sold over 125,000 copies in English and are being translated into 17 languages. In these books, I recommended that dieters choose whatever healthy, nutritious diet they wanted. I concentrated on providing readers with the thinking and behavioral skills they need to stay on their selected diet. Since the publication of these books, I have received valuable feedback from thousands of dieters who read the books or attended my workshops, as well as from comments I read online in blogs and in virtual communities.

I have learned a great deal from these dieters. First, I found that most dieters need more guidance in selecting their food. They just don't know how to select foods that minimize hunger and cravings. They don't know how to eat in a highly nutritious way. They don't know exactly what "balanced" means. Although they are able to stay within a reasonable calorie range, at least temporarily, they frequently do so in a way that isn't sufficiently healthy or sustainable in the long run. For example, they rarely eat enough protein and fiber, or they include too many high-fat, high-sugar foods. In addition, I found that many dieters don't count *all* of the calories they consume. They "forget" about the cream in their coffee, the olive oil on their vegetables, or the extra mayo in their tuna salad.

Some dieters run into trouble trying to apply to real life whichever eating plan they are following. They overeat at restaurants, social gatherings, family dinners, and special events. I also discovered that some readers simply are not using all of the skills I taught them to stay on the diet they selected. They institute the techniques they like—and ignore others. Or they use the skills, but not every day.

Based on this feedback, I modified my program. I changed how I taught certain skills, and I engaged a registered dietitian to help me fine-tune a food plan based on the eating choices of the most successful dieters I have counseled. The result is the book you hold in your hands. Throughout the pages of this book, you will learn and practice the skills you need so that *this time* you can lose weight forever.

By following the Beck Diet for Life Program in this book, you will evolve. You will stop the cycle of losing weight ... regaining ... losing weight ... regaining. I want you to know that *it isn't your fault* that you have not been able to break this cycle before now. It certainly isn't because you are weak or incapable of keeping off excess weight. To be a successful dieter and maintainer, you have to learn to follow a highly nutritious diet, use good eating habits, and refrain from eating food you haven't planned in advance to eat. To accomplish these three objectives, you have to learn to change your thinking. When you have such thoughts as, *It's okay if I eat this [unplanned food],* you will need to be ready with a strong response: *No, it's not okay—not if I want to lose weight and keep it off ... If I get involved with something else right now, my desire to eat this will fade away.* Throughout this book, you will learn to identify the thinking that is likely to derail you, and you will practice strong responses to these thoughts—over and over again.

Here is my best advice to you: Practice every skill I teach you in this book. Don't skip any. Give each exercise your best shot. It would be such a shame if you let your unhelpful thinking get in the way and prevent you from achieving permanent weight loss! If you do as I suggest, I'm sure you, too, will discover what the dieters I've counseled have discovered: It is so worth the effort to master every skill. It is worth the improved self-esteem, the better health, and the enriched life you will enjoy. It's worth the renewed confidence and control. It's worth the rest of your life!

*************

I hope you'll periodically visit www.beckdietforlife.com for information and inspiration, and I would so appreciate feedback on this book or my other books. You can contact me via the Web site.

# Part 1

# chapter 1

# Begin a New Way of Life

Visualize a day in the future: You wake up feeling refreshed. You get on the scale. It shows you're down another pound! You feel great. You get dressed in new clothes because your old ones are now too big. Friends, family, and coworkers have noticed the physical and psychological changes in you, and they often compliment you. You feel wonderful—you are energetic, and your health has improved.

Later that day, you return home from a party. It's the same annual party you attended last year, when you ate everything in sight and came home feeling upset and defeated. Today was different. You have changed. You haven't just lost weight. You have learned how to be a successful dieter. You are motivated, confident, and in control. And you know how to stay that way.

Why was your behavior at this year's party different? Because, this time, you went to the party with a plan. You fully enjoyed the food you ate and didn't feel guilty or lose control of your eating. Whenever you were tempted by food you hadn't planned in advance to eat, you stood firm. You told yourself, *No, it's not what I planned to eat, and I'd so much rather be thinner than have the momentary pleasure of eating this food,* and you were done with it. You didn't argue with yourself. You didn't struggle. You didn't say to yourself, *Oh, come on ... It's a special occasion ... It's just a little bit; it won't hurt.* You made a decision, and you easily stuck to it because you had the confidence to know you could. You enjoyed yourself, too, and you left feeling happy—happy that your clothes didn't feel tight, happy that the scale wouldn't go up the next day, happy that you spent your time socializing and having a good time instead of obsessing about food.

Not only did you stick to your eating plan at the party, but also you stuck to it all day long. If you had any cravings, you didn't pay much attention to them. If you were hungry and it wasn't mealtime or snack time, you easily said to yourself, *This is just hunger ... It's no big deal ... I'll just wait until it's time to eat.* At every snack and meal, you enjoyed every bite of your food.

You can make this scenario come true for you. You will learn a specific set of skills to enable you to follow the highly nutritious eating plan I provide for you in this book—in any situation. You will gain control of your eating at restaurants, buffets, and special events, as well as when traveling, on vacation, on weekends, and during holidays. You will learn what to do when you are stressed, tired, sick, upset, bored, or at loose ends. Not only will you gain control over your eating and weight, but in doing so you will also be more in control of your life.

That's what *The Complete Beck Diet for Life* does for you—it gives you your life back in so many ways:

- It frees you from guilt, worry, self-consciousness, and self-blame.

- It frees you from your fear of hunger and your fear of losing control.

- It frees you from overwhelming temptation and emotional eating.

- It frees you from feelings of deprivation, unfairness, and discouragement.

- It frees you from obsession about your food choices, weight, and appearance.

*The Complete Beck Diet for Life* is different from every other diet book you have read. It not only guides you in what to eat and how to eat, but also it helps you *change your mindset about dieting.* It leads you to make the psychological changes you need to be satisfied with your food choices, your ultimate weight, and yourself. Other diet plans focus exclusively on food. But they don't teach you what you need to do to follow the plan, day after day, no matter what the situation. This book is your instruction manual for motivating yourself for life.

My healthy eating plan teaches you how to maximize low-calorie filling foods— foods that are rich in protein, fiber, and healthy fats, as well as those that are low in sugar, refined starch, and unhealthy fats. These foods will help you feel full after eating fewer calories, so you won't have to battle the overwhelming hunger you may have experienced on other diets. My plan also teaches you how to include your favorite foods, as often as every day.

By following my plan, you will lose excess weight—and not just temporarily (for swimsuit season, a reunion, a wedding). Instead, you will lose it *for life*. And won't it be wonderful when you finally, really and truly, feel in control of your food choices, exercise habits, and weight?

With the Beck Diet for Life Program, you will successfully overcome common dieting challenges. Many diets ignore or gloss over the difficulties of dieting. They allege that you will not experience deprivation, hunger, or cravings. You have undoubtedly found that these kinds of claims are false. While the eating plan in this book minimizes hunger, deprivation, and cravings, no diet can eliminate them entirely. But you will learn exactly what to do when you experience these uncomfortable feelings. You will overcome these problems, learn from them, and actually use them to your advantage to build confidence, control, and strength.

## How the Program Works

There are several essential parts of the Beck Diet for Life Program. It provides you with a well-balanced, healthy, enjoyable eating plan. But before you change what you eat, you learn important skills:

- How to motivate yourself every day, make dieting a priority, give yourself credit, and cope with hunger and cravings

- How to consistently use good eating habits: eating everything slowly, while sitting down and enjoying every bite

- How to plan in advance what you are going to eat, monitor your eating as you go along, and stick with three meals and three snacks a day

You learn these skills as well as *how to get yourself to practice them,* day after day—even if you are tired, stressed, busy, or unmotivated. You learn how to exert self-control.

### On the Beck Diet for Life Program ...

You will learn to eat healthfully. You will develop an eating plan that you can comfortably stay on for life. The menus include such family favorites as meatloaf, chili, pizza, pasta, burgers, stir-fry, sandwiches, and much more. Some dishes require no cooking whatsoever, with many others going from refrigerator to table in 20 minutes or less. I have also used simple ingredients that you can find in any grocery store for a reasonable price. This is a diet you can easily enjoy and sustain—and it's not only good for you, but also good for your entire family.

**You will eat and fully enjoy your favorite foods and beverages.** This plan allows you to select—every day, if you wish—a reasonable portion of chips, fries, desserts, alcohol, or any other food or beverage you like. I will show you the portion you can eat and still lose weight, and I will teach you how to limit yourself to only that portion. Many of the dieters I counsel report that they are finally able to eat these formerly "forbidden" foods without guilt or fear—and each bite tastes that much better because they know they will feel satisfied, will easily limit themselves, and can have more the next day if they plan in advance.

**You will build confidence in your ability to follow a healthy diet and exercise plan.** Many dieters overwhelm themselves by trying to make too many changes at once. Instead, you will master one dieting skill at a time. You will learn what to say to yourself to ensure that you practice your new skills every day. You will prove to yourself over and over again that *you can get yourself to do what you need to do.* When dieting gets harder, you won't give up. You will keep on going because you will have learned the skills you need to navigate the tough times. You will know how to stay in control, no matter what. And even when you slip up, you will recover right away because you know what to do and have the confidence that you can exert the self-control to do it.

**You will turn mistakes into opportunities.** When unsuccessful dieters eat something they shouldn't, they tell themselves, *Now I've done it! I've really blown it ... Oh, well, I might as well eat whatever I want and start again tomorrow.* They may then eat hundreds or thousands of extra calories that day—or over the course of the next several days—and gain weight. This plan provides you with a Cheat Sheet (page 104), a worksheet that helps you recommit *immediately* whenever you make a mistake. From now on, your mistakes will not turn into an entire day or week of overeating, and you will learn how to avoid this kind of mistake in the future. The more times you get back on track immediately, the more you prove to yourself that you *can* do it—and it gets easier and easier to do so. Instead of becoming demoralized and hopeless, you will become a stronger and more confident dieter.

**You will maintain your weight loss.** I always tell dieters, "No wonder you always gained back weight in the past. You never learned the skills to keep it off." On this plan, you will learn how to motivate yourself every day, get back on track when you falter, and recover quickly from a relapse.

The Beck Diet for Life Program includes a plan for healthy eating. You already know that certain foods—vegetables, fruits, whole grains, beans, nuts, legumes—are much healthier selections than others, such as sweets, chips, and fried foods. The problems that beset most dieters: How to continually choose foods from the first category and limit (but not eliminate) foods from the second? How to get to the point where self-imposed restrictions feel good?

That is where Cognitive Therapy (sometimes called Cognitive Behavior Therapy) comes in. It is the most highly researched and effective form of talk therapy in the world. You will learn a powerful set of psychological tools that will enable you to stick to your healthy eating plan, no matter what. You will learn how to talk back to your inner saboteur, that voice that says:

> *It's okay [to stray from my diet] because ... I'm stressed ... I'm celebrating ... I'm tired ... I'm busy ... I really want it ... everyone else is eating it ... it's free ... it's only a little piece ... I deserve it ... it's a special occasion ... it won't matter ... I hardly ever get to have it ... I'll make up for it later.*

Have you had such thoughts? These "sabotaging thoughts" are common to any dieter who has struggled with losing weight or maintaining a weight loss. Cognitive Therapy teaches you to talk back to these thoughts in a convincing way. If you think, *I'll make up for it later,* you'll remind yourself, *When has "making up for it later" ever worked in the past? When has this idea ever helped me lose weight and keep it off?* Or if you think, *I really want that—it looks so good,* you will be able to firmly tell yourself: *This is just a desire to eat ... I'm not even hungry ... As soon as I turn my attention to something else, I won't even want it anymore ... I'm not going to eat it ... and I'm going to be so glad in a few minutes that I didn't.*

And you will be done with it.

First developed by my father, Aaron T. Beck, M.D., in the 1960s, Cognitive Therapy has been shown to help people overcome eating disorders, addictions, depression, anxiety, and many other psychological problems. Over 20 years ago, I started adapting the principles of Cognitive Therapy to help people achieve permanent weight loss. I lost 15 pounds along the way and have kept it off ever since. My patients and I don't worry that we will gain back weight because now we have the formula for success. We know exactly what to do.

Many dieters tell me that they can't lose weight because they have a slow metabolism, that they eat relatively little but still can't lose weight. As it turns out, they rarely have a medical problem that impedes weight loss. But they do have *thinking* problems. For example, they think they should restrict themselves severely to lose weight quickly (not realizing that their bodies will rebel and that they will then overeat). Dieters think that somehow calories don't count if they eat while standing up, cooking, or clearing the table, or when no one is watching. They think that it is legitimate to deviate from their plan (and that somehow they won't gain weight) as long as they can think of a "good" reason: *I'm out to dinner ... It's a holiday ... My day is so stressful, I feel like letting loose.* They think it is "bad" and "abnormal" to feel hungry. They think it's necessary to bulk up at meals or carry food with them to avoid hunger. They think if they make one mistake, they should give up and wait until the next day to start again—and eat whatever they want until then.

When dieters first come to see me, they invariably have unhealthful eating habits. Sometimes they eat too quickly, without being fully aware of what they are eating, and they don't enjoy every bite. Sometimes they eat moderately in front of others and then eat out of hand when no one is around. They often eat when they just feel like eating, even if they are not actually hungry. For example, they eat when they are bored, upset, celebrating, or procrastinating; when someone offers them something to eat; when they smell delicious food; when they see a food commercial; when they prepare meals; and when they clean up after meals. When they "cheat," they tend to quickly devour food, trying not to notice how much they are eating to avoid feeling guilty.

As it turns out, all of the dieters I have worked with ate more—and in some cases a great deal more—than they initially realized. They just were not fully aware of the extent of their overeating. Once they learned how to change their thinking about eating, they were able to slow down, really notice everything they were eating, enjoy their food without guilt, and—finally—stick to a diet. Rather than having good eating days and bad eating days, they learned to eat consistently every day.

Researchers have demonstrated that Cognitive Therapy works for eating disorders—and for weight loss. In a Swedish study of 54 women, participants who enrolled in a Cognitive Therapy weight-loss program for just 10 sessions lost an average of nearly 19 pounds, compared with an average of just 1.5 pounds for study participants who received advice about exercise and other weight-loss behaviors but did not learn essential Cognitive Therapy techniques. A year and a half after the end of the program, the participants in the Cognitive Therapy group maintained most of their weight loss (keeping off an average of 13 pounds), whereas the non-Cognitive Therapy group gained weight, ending up *heavier* than they were before the study began.

A previous study by the same Swedish researchers of 105 men and women determined that study participants in a Cognitive Therapy group lost an average of

18 pounds over 10 weeks and continued to lose weight after their counseling sessions ended, losing an average of 22 pounds in 18 months. Participants who were not in the Cognitive Therapy group *gained* an average of 5 pounds during the same time period.

## You Will Change Your Mindset

By the time you finish the Beck Diet for Life Program, you will notice how different the "new" you is from the "old" you.

**The old you thought:** *I'm hungry. I have to eat.*
**The new you thinks:** *I'm hungry. Oh, well, dinner is in an hour. I'll wait.*

**The old you thought:** *I'm upset. I need to eat.*
**The new you thinks:** *I'm upset. If I eat, I'll feel even worse. I'll go calm myself down using the new techniques I've learned.*

**The old you thought:** *It won't matter if I eat this unplanned food because it's only a small piece.*
**The new you thinks:** *It does matter. If I eat this, I'll be strengthening my giving-in habit.*

**The old you thought:** *Uh-oh, I might lose control and eat too much at the party.*
**The new you thinks:** *I know exactly what to do if I'm tempted.*

**The old you thought:** *I have to eat this unplanned food my hostess is offering.*
**The new you thinks:** *I'll politely say, "No, thanks," because I'm entitled to stick up for myself, even if my hostess is momentarily disappointed.*

**The old you thought:** *I can eat on the fly.*
**The new you thinks:** *NO CHOICE. I have to take the time I need to buy food, prepare it, and eat it slowly, enjoying every bite.*

**The old you thought:** *There are "good" foods and "bad" foods. I should never have a bad food.*
**The new you thinks:** *I can eat a favorite food, in a reasonable portion, as often as once a day.*

**The old you thought:** *I just cheated on my diet. I've blown it. I may as well continue eating whatever I want and start again tomorrow.*
**The new you thinks:** *Okay, I made a mistake. No big deal. I'll start again right this minute so I won't gain weight.*

**The old you thought:** *This is too hard. I'm giving up.*
**The new you thinks:** *It feels hard right at the moment, but this feeling is temporary. I'll go distract myself and in a few minutes, I'll be really glad I did.*

*The old you thought: I'm just a weak person where food and dieting are concerned.*
*The new you thinks: I know that if I keep practicing these skills, I will gain control.*
*I'm learning how to be strong.*

How will you achieve this transformation? I'll teach you!

## Get Ready to Strengthen Your Resistance Muscle

To lose weight permanently, you need Cognitive Therapy techniques to develop a powerful "resistance muscle," a psychological muscle that you flex whenever you stand firm and stick to the program. This muscle gives you the ability to do what you need to do to lose weight permanently.

Every single time you say no to unplanned food, you fortify your resistance muscle, which makes it more likely that you will be able to resist the next time … and the time after that … and the time after that. Every time you don't feel like practicing a skill but you do it anyway, you strengthen your resistance muscle, which makes it easier and easier to get yourself to practice your skills in the future.

On the other hand, every time you eat something you hadn't planned to eat, you weaken your resistance muscle and strengthen your "giving-in" muscle. When you say yes to unplanned food, even if you're eating only crumbs, you make it more likely that you will give in the next time … and the time after that … and the time after that. This is why every single bite of unplanned food matters. It's not just the calories; *it's the habit*. Every time you skip practicing a skill, you strengthen your giving-in muscle and make it less likely that you will consistently use that skill in the future. So every time matters.

The more you build your resistance muscle and weaken your giving-in muscle, the easier and easier dieting becomes. You are offered a piece of chocolate, and you spontaneously say, "No, thanks," because you are thinking, *I'd rather be thinner.* You are tempted to take a second slice of bread from the restaurant basket, but you automatically reject the idea: *No, I didn't plan to have it.* If you are tempted to take the partial cookie left on a tray in the office kitchen, you think, *No, I'm not going to have it … Remember yesterday when I turned down the coffee cake, and I felt really good about it? I did it then, so I know I can do it now.* You don't struggle. It isn't painful to turn down food because you've proven to yourself over and over that you can. And not only do you have the confidence to know you can turn down food, but also you know that you feel so much better when you do—strong, confident, and in control. Life becomes so much easier when your resistance muscle is strong.

You strengthen your resistance muscle just as you would strengthen any muscle in your body—by using it over and over. If you want to strengthen your biceps, you lift weights, starting with relatively light dumbbells and progressing to heavier ones as your arm muscles get stronger. It's the same with your resistance muscle: In Stage 1, you will start out "light" as you strengthen your resistance while still eating your usual foods. In Stage 2, you will increase your resistance as you transition to the Think Thin Initial Eating Plan and eat in the controlled environment of your home. In Stage 3, you will strengthen it even more by increasing the challenge yet again, by learning how to resist temptation in more difficult situations, such as restaurants and social occasions. By Stage 4, you will have strengthened your resistance muscle enough to adopt the more flexible Think Thin Lifetime Eating Plan. In Stage 5, you will learn how to continue to use your resistance muscle throughout your life.

## The Role of Thinking

Some dieters erroneously believe that they can't develop a strong resistance muscle because they think they eat "automatically." They say they don't know how they finished the box of crackers or the bag of trail mix. But eating is never automatic. Digestion is automatic. The beating of your heart is automatic. Eating is not.

Before you eat, you always have a thought, even if you're not fully conscious of it. The thought may be as simple as, *I'm going to eat this.* The Beck Diet for Life Program teaches you how to recognize these kinds of thoughts, especially the sabotaging thoughts that encourage you to eat unplanned food. They often start with:

- *It's okay to eat [this unplanned food] because....*

- *It won't matter if I eat [this unplanned food] because....*

You have probably experienced lots of sabotaging thoughts in the past. Because you didn't know how to recognize or respond to them, these thoughts eventually led you to stray from your diet or abandon it altogether. The Beck Diet for Life Program teaches you how to talk back to these thoughts, so that you stand firm and exercise your resistance muscle. If you don't learn how to talk back to your sabotaging thoughts, you will give in, eat, and weaken your resistance muscle.

You will learn how to talk back to these thoughts by making Response Cards, which are index cards (or the equivalent) with important reminders that you read every day. You will rehearse the ideas in your Response Cards over and over again

**Change your thinking,** and you can change your behavior permanently. **Change your behavior,** and weight loss will follow.

to prepare yourself for challenging situations. For example, at some point you will have a thought such as, *I don't care ... I know I'm not supposed to have this brownie, but I'm going to have it anyway.* You will then pull out a Response Card that you have been reading every day that says:

> It is true that I don't care at this very moment. But if I eat this unplanned food, I am going to care quite a lot in just a few minutes. I know I will feel really bad if I give in, but I will feel terrific if I resist. I need to go do something else!

Eventually, the messages on your Response Cards will become ingrained. You will build new pathways in your mind, so when you experience sabotaging thoughts, you will automatically answer them without thinking too much about it. Once you get to this point, sticking to your diet gets dramatically easier. That's when you will breathe a sigh of relief. You will know the formula works for you, too. That's when you will realize that dieting is worth it—so worth it. *That's the moment when you start to get your life back.*

# chapter 2

# Experience the Difference

I t doesn't matter how many times you have tried to lose excess weight in the past or how many collective pounds you have lost and then regained. This really can be the last time you ever need to lose weight. *Ever*. This time will be different.

I know, you have probably said those same last five words to yourself many times. You probably said them just before you started your last diet. Maybe you lost some weight but gained it back. If going on the last diet wasn't different, why should you believe me when I tell you that this time will be? *Because I know why you struggled.* Other diet programs didn't teach you what you need to know for lifetime weight-loss success. The Beck Diet for Life Program gives you those skills.

You may not have known this before, but successful dieting requires a set of skills, and it takes instruction and practice to master them and use them consistently. No one expects to be able to sit behind the wheel of a car for the very first time and drive perfectly. No one expects to pick up a musical instrument and play it well before taking lessons and practicing. Yet nearly everyone expects to be able to follow a diet immediately, without learning anything new and certainly without practicing dieting skills. One of the reasons this time will be different is because I am going to teach you these skills, *and* I'm going to teach you how to get yourself to *practice* them day after day.

This time is going to be different because the Beck Diet for Life Program is different. Here is how:

**It teaches you how to satisfy your hunger.** Did you know that some foods decrease hunger and cravings and other foods actually increase them? To achieve sustained weight loss, it is not just a matter of calories in, energy out. It's what makes up those calories, because the composition of those calories makes a big difference. Many diets let you select foods that don't allow you to eat in a healthful, well-balanced way. The Think Thin Eating Plans teach you the formula that maximizes fullness and sound nutrition.

**It teaches you how to include your favorite foods.** You have likely tried diets that outright banned certain foods and beverages, such as sweets, chips, and alcohol. While it is true that you can't consume large portions of these items and still lose weight, you *can* eat limited amounts of at least one favorite food every single day. You will be able to satisfy your taste for indulgences and not feel the need to go overboard because you will know that you can always plan to have more tomorrow.

**It teaches you how to be satisfied with less.** Do you sometimes wolf down your food, hardly noticing what you are eating? This program will teach you how to slow down and enjoy every bite that you eat. Have you felt deprived when you saw other people eating food you knew you weren't supposed to eat? This program teaches you a new mindset. It helps you see that you will either be deprived of some amount of food or you will be deprived of losing weight, feeling better about yourself, being healthier, fitting into smaller-sized clothing, and all of the other wonderful benefits of being thinner.

**It teaches you what to do when you want to eat, but it's not time to eat.** People want to eat for lots of reasons. They want to eat when they are hungry, craving, stressed, tired, bored, upset, celebrating, or procrastinating. They want to eat when they smell food cooking, when they see a food commercial, or when they pass by a bakery. The Beck Diet for Life Program teaches you what to say to yourself in these situations and what to do to avoid consuming extra calories.

**It teaches you how to stay motivated.** If you are like most dieters, you feel motivated during the initial weeks of any diet. But you don't know what to do when your motivation inevitably wanes. On this program, you will learn to motivate yourself every day through a number of techniques. You will continually rehearse the reasons you want to lose weight. You will give yourself credit for every positive eating behavior you use. You will create a Memory Box to store your positive diet-related memories: how terrific you felt the first time you successfully conquered a craving;

how wonderful it was to buy clothing in smaller sizes; or how pleased you were when you received special compliments. You will read these positive memories often to remind yourself that it's worth mastering and using these skills.

**It teaches you how to get back on track.** It is normal to stray from your diet. I know you will make mistakes. That is why you will practice in advance what to do when you fall off the wagon, so you can get back on *right away*—not tomorrow, next week, or next month. You will learn how to continually and quickly recommit yourself to the program and reduce the likelihood of making mistakes in the future.

**It teaches you how to keep going when dieting gets tough.** Like all dieters, you will find that it is easy to diet on some days and harder on others. This is normal. It becomes more difficult, for example, when you are struggling with negative emotions, tired, or tempted to skip exercising or shopping for and preparing the food you need. It gets harder when your hormones are fluctuating and your cravings for certain foods intensify. It gets harder as life presents challenges at work or at home and as the rate you are losing weight starts to slow. In this program, you will not only learn but also you will actually *master* a set of thinking skills to prevent yourself from getting discouraged and abandoning your diet when times get tough. You will prove to yourself—over and over—that these difficult days always pass and that you're always so glad later you stuck with it.

**It teaches you how to maintain your new weight.** Knowing how to keep off the weight you lose also requires a special set of skills, such as knowing how to become a more flexible eater and how to continue to motivate yourself every day, even after the number on the scale has stopped going down. I've found that many people who lose weight simply forget what it felt like to be overweight, taking their new weight—and all of the benefits they have achieved—for granted. Once they stop feeling as if watching their weight is worth it, they start gaining. Then they feel panicky and hopeless. I'll teach you how to always remember why you wanted to lose weight in the first place and why it's worth it to continue working at keeping it off.

The Beck Diet for Life Program can help you in other ways, too, since I have found that dieters often derive unexpected benefits. For example, you can:

**Learn how to get yourself to do other tasks you tend to avoid.** Many dieters have told me that they've used the skills in this plan to accomplish numerous tasks, such as sticking to a budget, being more productive at work, maintaining a more organized household, and doing self-care activities. As you better organize yourself for dieting and maintaining, you will learn to better organize your life—period.

**Become a more assertive person.** You will learn how to make time in your schedule to eat properly, ask for what you need at restaurants, and nicely turn down offers to eat unplanned food. You will feel entitled to get your needs met, even if it means disappointing or inconveniencing someone else. Many dieters find that they spontaneously apply their newly developed skills to assert themselves in other areas of their lives, too.

**Free up time and energy to live your life.** Many dieters spend an enormous amount of time thinking about food. They fear getting on the scale. They feel bad about their appearance and about themselves. They are afraid others will judge them negatively. They are embarrassed to eat in public. They feel despondent when they gain weight. The Beck Diet for Life Program helps you get in control—so that you will no longer obsess about food or your body, or feel guilty or embarrassed. In doing so, you will have more physical and mental energy. You will feel proud, in control, and optimistic about the future.

* * * * * * * * * * * * *

That's just a taste of why this time is different. It's different because this time, over the coming weeks and months, I'm going to teach you how to overcome the problems that have blocked you from achieving your goal of lasting weight loss. I'll teach you how to do this in small, achicvable steps that span five stages. Here's a brief preview of the important dieting skills you will learn in each stage.

# Stage 1

To start out, you will learn and practice nine Success Skills adapted from the most successful dieters I've counseled. You will master these skills—such as continually motivating yourself, weighing yourself daily, eating slowly, and overcoming hunger and cravings—*before* you transition to the Think Thin Initial Eating Plan in Stage 2.

Many dieters don't want to wait to start a diet because they want to start losing weight this very moment. I will give you a few minor ways to change your eating at the beginning of Stage 1. But I have found—over and over again—that it is just too overwhelming to stick to a comprehensive eating plan while still learning such essential skills as eating everything slowly, while sitting down and enjoying every bite. Sure, you can lose excess weight without learning these skills. You have undoubtedly done so in the past. But you haven't been able to keep it off.

I find that dieters who try to do too much at once don't master the Sucess Skills and end up failing sooner or later. I say to dieters who are in too much of a rush, "You have already done the experiment of jumping into dieting. Has it worked for you long term?" Obviously it hasn't, or they wouldn't need my help. This question makes them more motivated to hold off on starting the Think Thin Initial Eating Plan until they have mastered the skills they need.

I also give them the following analogy: Trying to change what you eat without first learning these dieting skills is like trying to drive a car on a busy street after only one lesson in a parking lot. You may be able to drive out of the lot, but as soon as you get into traffic on a busy street, you're in trouble. You don't know how to safely change lanes or use your mirrors to avoid blind spots. You don't yet have the judgment to know how closely you can drive next to other cars. You get scared or fed up. You think, *I can't do this ... It's too hard,* and you're ready to give up driving altogether.

If you are like most people when they start a diet, you take a similar approach: You try to go from 0 to 60 within seconds. You even manage to lose a few pounds before you start to encounter obstacles. The flat tires, rainstorms, potholes, and detours of dieting come in the form of social gatherings, restaurant meals, strong negative emotions, cravings, hunger, and more. If you don't learn the skills you need to follow your diet no matter which obstacles you face—*before* you encounter them—you will eventually lose your way, mentally wave a white towel in the air in defeat, and walk away from the diet. Worse, you are likely to emerge from the experience disappointed and less confident than when you started, making it that much harder to try again.

Once you learn and practice the Success Skills, you will have a much easier time standing firm in the face of dieting challenges. You will know what to do when you feel hungry but it's not time to eat. You will know what to say to yourself to resist the treats coworkers bring to office meetings. You will know how to ride out a craving and how to prioritize dieting no matter how busy your life becomes. When your family members try to cajole you into taking second helpings at a holiday meal or undermine your progress, you will know what to tell them.

You will always be faced with tempting foods that you have to limit. Wouldn't it be wonderful to find it easy to resist? If so, you have to learn and practice the Success Skills over and over again. These skills are so important that you will not only use them during Stage 1, but also you will continue to practice and brush up on them in every subsequent stage—and to use some of them for the rest of your life.

# Stage 2

Once you master the Success Skills, you're ready to start the Think Thin Initial Eating Plan. This is a nutritious diet that provides the basis for the Think Thin Lifetime Eating Plan, which, as the name implies, you can use for life. You will stick with the plan because:

**You will enjoy real food, not "diet" food.** The Think Thin Initial Eating Plan includes an assortment of meal options that are rich in fiber, lean protein, and other important nutrients. These options also include real foods that real people like to eat—such as pizza, soups, steak, lasagna, spaghetti and meatballs, and more. These are foods you can feel good about feeding yourself and your family. It's simple food, too. You won't have to spend lots of time and energy learning new recipes or cooking techniques—unless you really want to. And it's convenient. I've even included healthful no-cook options.

**You won't make any food off-limits.** I don't believe in forbidden foods for two main reasons: First, I think you should be able to enjoy any food in moderation. Second, putting foods on a "never eat" list puts you at risk of going way overboard whenever you invariably end up eating them anyway.

There's a better way—one that is much more delicious and satisfying. On the Think Thin Initial Eating Plan, you will gain confidence and control by allowing yourself a reasonable portion of any desired treat as often as once a day. Every day you will have 150 or 200 Bonus Calories to spend on any food or beverage that you wish, such as chips, pretzels, sweets, desserts, or alcohol. You can't eat whichever food or beverage you want in whatever quantity you want, whenever you want it. If you did, you would, of course, gain weight. But you can *plan* to eat limited amounts of your favorites every day.

**You will know what to do when you reach a plateau.** You will select from one of five balanced, calorie-controlled plans, based on your current activity level, gender, age, height, and weight. As you lose excess weight, you will step down from a higher-calorie plan to a lower-calorie one, cutting no more than 200 daily calories at a time to prevent a decrease in your metabolism. You will lose weight in a sustainable way. And each time you plateau, you will decide whether it's worth it to lower your calorie level again.

**You won't feel as hungry as you have on other diets.** The Think Thin plan satisfies hunger because, at every eating opportunity, you will consume a mixture of the following three filling nutrients.

**Lean Protein:** I've found time and time again that whenever dieters skimp on protein, they're ravenous between meals. Research clearly shows that consuming more protein can minimize hunger. Consider the following:

- In a University of Minnesota study of 40 people, study participants more quickly lost their desire to eat when they snacked on yogurt fortified with whey protein compared with a lower-protein yogurt. The same was true when study participants ate a ham sandwich for lunch compared with a bacon sandwich (which is lower in protein).

- In a Purdue University study of 46 women, participants who followed a higher-protein diet (30 percent protein) felt more satisfied than women on a lower-protein diet (18 percent protein).

You will choose from a wide variety of protein-rich foods, including beef, poultry, pork, fish, shellfish, beans, dairy products, and tofu.

**Quality Carbohydrates:** You will consume high-quality carbohydrates from whole grains, legumes, nuts, vegetables, and fruits. These foods are rich in vitamins, minerals, plant nutrients, and fiber—all of which are important for total body health. Fiber, in particular, makes weight loss easier. Like protein, it reduces hunger and increases satisfaction. It does so in the following ways:

- Fiber-rich foods tend to be chewy, which slows the pace of eating, allowing more time for the "I'm full" message from your stomach to reach your brain.

- Your body can't digest and absorb dietary fiber. It passes through your gastrointestinal tract intact. It fills you up and allows you to experience the pleasure of eating—you can chew it, swallow it, and feel it fill up your stomach—but it doesn't load you up with lots of calories.

- High-fiber foods are relatively heavy, helping to trigger feelings of fullness by weighing down your stomach and triggering stretch receptors that relay the "I'm full" message to your brain.

- Fiber slows digestion. Your body breaks down all carbohydrates into sugars (called glucose) that are eventually absorbed into your bloodstream. Fiber mixes with partially digested food contents in the intestines, creating a thick gel that slows the absorption of glucose into the bloodstream. This not only provides you with slow-release energy, but also it reduces hunger.

For all of those reasons and more, people who include more fiber in their diets tend to eat fewer overall calories. A Tufts University study determined that eating an additional 14 grams of fiber daily—roughly double the amount most people consume—reduces eating by 10 percent. And fiber's appetite-suppressing effect seems to be more potent the more overweight a person is. In studies that included only obese participants, doubling the amount of daily fiber grams suppressed eating by 18 percent—that's enough to trigger a 5-pound weight loss over nearly 4 months.

**Fat:** The Think Thin plan includes modest amounts of fatty foods, which help fill you up, make food taste good, and add to your satisfaction. Some fatty foods—such as olives, nuts, avocado, and certain kinds of oil—contain a specific type of fat, called monounsaturated fat, that is thought to help improve health.

> ## What Is a Balanced Meal?
>
> Many dieters wonder why they feel hungry shortly after a meal. Usually it's because they eat too fast (and don't give their brain enough time to register fullness) or they don't consume their calories wisely. They often eat too many low-quality carbohydrates. They might eat just pasta or pizza, for instance, or a sandwich with too much bread and too little meat. A balanced meal that contains lean protein, vegetables, high-quality carbohydrates, and a little bit of fat will make you feel much more satisfied.

**You will continue to eat this way for a lifetime.** You don't go on this diet and then go off of it. You go on it, adapt it until it's comfortable and easy, and you *stay* on it—breaking the cycle of yo-yo dieting and achieving permanent weight loss. That's yet another way this eating plan is different. You won't stick exclusively to the limited options in Stage 2 for long. And in Stage 4, I'll teach you how to modify the plan to include your personal recipes. I'll also teach you how and when to make flexible rules for eating, so that you will continue to benefit from the diet forever, without regaining the weight you lose. In short, I'll provide you with the eating plan that you can stick with for life.

# Stage 3

Many people blame our epidemic of obesity on the rise in highly caloric, highly palatable convenience foods. They point out that restaurant portions have grown by up to 60 percent in the past two decades, in step with rising numbers of overweight and obese adults.

The truth of the matter is that highly processed foods and large restaurant portions are not going to disappear. Neither are fast-food joints, all-you-can-eat buffets, or cafeterias. To lose excess weight and keep it off, you will learn how to stay in control in any eating situation, including at restaurants, parties, and extended family dinners. You will learn how to stay in control when you are stressed, sick, busy, or traveling. These challenging situations simply require a set of dieting skills—skills that will build on what you will already have learned during Stage 1.

# Stage 4

By the time you enter this stage, you will have fully strengthened your resistance muscle. You will be able to quickly get back on track whenever you make a mistake. You will no longer fear hunger or cravings. You will have transformed a feeling of deprivation into a sense of triumph and a feeling of unfairness about dieting into a sense that everything you need to do to lose weight—no matter how challenging—is worth it. You will know how to consistently make time for dieting, and you will know how to continually motivate yourself, too.

You will also be ready to start a transition into rest-of-your-life eating, starting with greater flexibility. You will experiment with skipping snacks and adding that food to meals or occasionally banking snack calories to splurge for a special dinner or larger-than-usual dessert. If you love a highly processed food (such as a lower-protein cereal or less-nutritious white bread) *and you miss eating it,* you will experiment with occasionally replacing healthier choices with these foods to see how they affect your hunger, cravings, and energy level. You will learn to use a basic formula to plan your meals and how to adapt your favorite recipes. You will customize the Think Thin Lifetime Eating Plan and make it your own.

# Stage 5

As you near maintenance, the initial thrill of dieting usually wears off. You don't see a drop in weight every week or maybe even every other week. You stay in the same clothing size for much longer. You start taking the many amazing benefits of weight loss for granted, and your motivation goes down.

In this stage, you will learn how to keep yourself motivated for life. With a Daily Motivation Plan, a Re-Motivation Plan, and a Get-Back-on-Track Plan, you will learn what to do if all of your efforts to lose weight and keep it off just don't seem worth it at the moment. Most important, you will learn what to do if you relapse, as well as how to prevent a relapse in the future.

\*\*\*\*\*\*\*\*\*\*\*\*\*\*

I hope you are now convinced that this approach is different. The work you put in at the beginning of this program will truly pay off in the end—and the payoff never ends. This time, you can go on to a lifetime of weight maintenance. You won't lose the weight just to regain it again, then go on yet another diet, and lose weight again. This time you will get thinner, stay thinner, feel good about yourself, have more self-confidence, and enjoy better health—for the rest of your life.

## *Is This Book for You?*

Please be sure to consult your health-care professional before starting the diet and exercise programs in this book to see whether they are right for you.

You should not follow the Beck Diet for Life Program if you suffer from an eating disorder, depression, anxiety, or other psychological problem. Work with a mental-health professional to resolve your difficulties *before* you start dieting. It is much too difficult to work on both simultaneously. To find a certified Cognitive Therapist near you, go to the Academy of Cognitive Therapy's Web site at www.academyofct.org.

You should also postpone starting this program if your life is just too busy and stressful right now. The program takes a strong commitment from you and initially requires a fair degree of time and energy (though as you master skills, it gets easier and easier). Reduce your stress and then start with a fresh mind and renewed energy.

# chapter 3

# Get Ready to Lose

Y ou are almost ready to start the Beck Diet for Life Program. In Stage 1, you will start learning and practicing the skills you will need for lifelong weight loss and maintenance.

Before you start, however, I would like you to do the following 10 essential tasks.

# task 1

### Gather Your Supplies

You will use a number of inexpensive, easy-to-find supplies over and over again while on this plan. You probably already have some of them. Gather the following:

- **A set of 3 x 5 index cards in any color.** You will use these to create Response Cards.

- **A set of blank business-sized cards.** You will use these cards to create your Advantages Deck, a special set of Response Cards that you will read daily to remind yourself why weight loss is so worth it. You can find these cards—some with decorative backgrounds—at office-supply stores or online.

- **A Diet Notebook.** You will use a bound notebook to write such important information as food plans, results of eating experiments, and notes to remember for the future.

- **A digital scale.** Preferably choose one that weighs to the half pound, so you can weigh yourself daily and keep track of your progress.

- **Graph paper.** You will use it to chart your weight loss.

- **A small box.** Select one about the size used to file recipe cards. You will turn this into a Memory Box (page 38) where you can store important weight-loss milestones and memories.

- **A larger box.** You will use this to store distractions to help wait out cravings, negative emotions, and other precipitants to unplanned eating.

- **Multiple sets of measuring spoons and cups.** You will be using these essentials several times a day. You will be less likely to measure your food if your only set is in the dishwasher, still dirty.

- **A digital food scale.** You will use this indispensable tool to accurately measure your food by weight.

- **Smaller plates and bowls (optional).** You will be more visually satisfied if your portions seem larger. If you get ½- and 1-cup bowls, you won't need to use measuring cups as often and you can eat directly from them, which will reduce cleanup time.

- **Smaller forks and spoons (optional).** These utensils will help you take smaller bites so your food will last longer. For the same reason, some dieters enjoy using chopsticks, regardless of which type of food they are eating.

# task 2
### Set a Modest Weight-Loss Goal

Perhaps you already have a specific number you want to hit on the scale. Or maybe you are aiming to fit into a specific clothing size. But you don't yet know whether your particular goal is realistic, and you may get discouraged by how long term that goal is. You will be better able to motivate yourself if you set a series of short-term goals instead.

Make your initial goal to lose just 5 pounds. University of Minnesota research shows that people with smaller short-term goals are more likely to achieve those goals and to maintain their weight loss long term. Once you reach your first 5-pound milestone, you can then set another goal to lose an additional 5 pounds ... and then another ... and then another.

I also want you to celebrate every time you reach a 5-pound milestone. Buy a new article of clothing or accessory. Get a new computer game, CD, or DVD. Treat yourself to a manicure, pedicure, or massage. Get tickets to an entertainment or sporting event. Buy a charm bracelet and get a new charm to commemorate each milestone. You can set whatever reward you want—as long as it doesn't involve food. Take a moment now to think how you will reward each 5-pound milestone. Write down a few ideas in your Diet Notebook under the heading "Rewards for Losing 5 Pounds."

# task 3
## Make Time for Dieting

Dieting requires a commitment. To lose weight successfully, dieting should be your top priority for a long time, and maintaining your new habits will always be high on your list if you want to keep off the excess weight for life. Many of the tasks I suggest you complete throughout this program don't take a great deal of time to do, but don't fool yourself into thinking that you will somehow be able to just find the time. You will have to plan precisely when you are going to do each task. Otherwise, you will find yourself making excuses, such as, *I don't have time* or *I'm too rushed.* Making excuses is a slippery slope that leads to failure.

To lose weight successfully, you will need time to:

- Read this book.

- Practice skills, such as planning and monitoring your food intake.

- Exercise regularly.

- Shop for food and prepare meals.

- Sit down for three meals and three snacks every day, eating all food slowly.

- Get enough sleep. Lack of sleep can lower your motivation and lead to overeating.

If your life is relatively calm and you are already good at following a schedule, it may not be difficult to set aside the time you need for yourself. If your schedule is already very full, however, you will have to decide which tasks and activities you will postpone, delegate, cut back on, or do less well—at least for the time being. I tell the dieters I counsel that it's impossible to add more water to an already full glass. If your glass is full, you have to spill some out before you can pour more in. You'll have to actively work to find the time you will need.

I want you to know that you won't always have to spend so much time and energy on dieting, but you *will* need to do so in the beginning. With practice, your new skills will become second nature, but even then you will periodically need to spend extra time and energy on dieting as you face life's challenges.

# reality check

**If you are thinking:** *I'll figure out how to squeeze in these diet and exercise activities when the time comes.*

**Face reality:** You're setting yourself up for failure. Extra time will not magically make itself available. You have to plan your life around diet and exercise activities—not vice versa.

# task 4

## Get a Diet Buddy

Successful dieters have a trusted friend, family member, or fellow dieter to help them with the challenges of dieting. If you are like many dieters, you are probably thinking, *No way am I telling anyone I'm on a diet.* I understand your concern. So many of the dieters I have counseled were initially so ashamed of their weight that they thought, *What if I fail again? I don't want anyone to know.*

The irony is that by *not* lining up support, you are making dieting even harder. Few dieters—especially chronic dieters—can achieve lasting weight loss without the help, encouragement, and accountability that only another person can provide. A University of North Carolina study of 192 dieters determined that dieters who regularly e-mailed a weight-loss counselor lost twice as much weight during a three-month period as dieters who had no e-mail support. In a study of 1,032 dieters completed by researchers from Duke University and researchers from a number of participating institutions, dieters who regularly contacted a counselor were much less likely to relapse and regain lost weight during a three-year period than dieters who did not have support.

A Diet Buddy helps keep you accountable. Unsuccessful dieters are very good at fooling themselves. They forget to practice every skill, weigh themselves daily (especially if they think the number on the scale has gone up), and count every calorie. They think they can be an effective dieter and maintainer if they do a "pretty good" job using their skills and following their eating plan, instead of doing a thorough and complete job. The most important task of a Diet Buddy is to help you make sure you are doing what you need to do *every day.*

You may even be able to find a Diet Buddy online, although I recommend that you persist in finding one with whom you can have voice-to-voice contact. Online communities are wonderful at supporting dieters, helping them solve problems, and getting them to realize that they are not alone in their struggles. But dieters can too easily fail to post on any given day, and they can post messages without reporting their change in weight and the skills they did—or didn't—do, depriving themselves of the key benefit of a Diet Buddy: accountability.

At the very least, you need to communicate with your Diet Buddy daily—either through phone calls (you can leave voice-mail messages), faxes, or e-mails—to report your change in weight (you don't need to reveal your actual weight), as well as how well you completed each task in the program. Report all of this information *first*. If you didn't practice a Success Skill (or didn't do it completely), tell your Diet Buddy your plan for how you *will* do it the next day—and consistently every day after that. Or ask for help in figuring out what to do. Your buddy can help you distinguish between unavoidable problems (you unexpectedly had to take your child to the doctor and didn't have time to get to the supermarket) versus avoidable problems (you knew your day would be busy, but you didn't figure out ahead of time when you would buy food).

It's easy to omit or gloss over your mistakes when you contact your Diet Buddy. That is why you should begin the conversation by reviewing the skills on your Success Skills Sheets (pages 266–275), which you will begin filling out when you start Stage 1 and continue to fill out for a very long time. Remember, the most important part of the communication with your Diet Buddy is to report on your progress and your mistakes and to get help with any problems you are having.

When you know you will have to give an honest report to another person, it is easier to respond to the sabotaging thought, *I think I'll skip practicing this skill today,* or, *It won't matter if I eat this unplanned food,* by telling yourself, *No, I'm not going to skip it,* or, *I'm not going to cheat because I don't want to have to tell my Diet Buddy.*

At a minimum, use your Diet Buddy to help keep you accountable. If you wish, a Diet Buddy can help even more: If you give him/her a copy of this book to read, your buddy can increase your sense of hope and help you give yourself credit for every positive eating behavior you engage in. A buddy can reduce your shame, reminding you that it's not your fault you had difficulty losing weight or keeping it off in the past. He/she can assure you that your weight is superficial—not who you are inside—and can help you stop judging yourself harshly. When dieting feels too hard, a buddy can remind you why it's worth it. He/she can help you come up with practical solutions to problems, such as finding time to exercise or prepare meals. Your buddy can point out additional benefits of weight loss that you might take for granted, as well as help you talk back to your sabotaging thoughts, create Response

Cards, and solve problems. He/she can help you put mistakes in perspective and talk you through difficult moments when temptation is great. In addition, your Diet Buddy can help keep you motivated, reminding you (when you have momentarily forgotten) why you had wholeheartedly committed yourself to following the Beck Diet for Life Program to lose excess weight.

Even if you're also seeking the help of a diet professional, I'd like you to have your own personal Diet Buddy whom you can call or e-mail every day, even on the spur of the moment when you need help—now and into the future.

# task 5
## Get Organized

The state of your kitchen and dining room can influence how you follow the Beck Diet for Life Program. If these rooms are cluttered and messy, it can make you feel out of control, which can affect your confidence in staying in control of your eating.

Following the program will be easier if you can readily find the dishes and utensils you need. As you rearrange them, look through your cabinets. What can you get rid of? Appliances, pots and pans, or dishes you never use? Food that is out of date?

Also look in your refrigerator and cabinets for foods that you might find overly tempting. On this program, you can eat a favorite food in a reasonable portion once a day. But initially some foods may be too difficult for you to have around. Seeing certain foods may trigger a strong desire to eat. For example, one study found that office workers ate more chocolate if they kept the candy on their desks rather than just 2 yards away. When candy was put in opaque jars, office workers consumed significantly less than when it was kept in clear jars. Eventually, you will find that you have an easier and easier time handling the various triggers that lead you to eat. For now, however, it is best to eliminate as many triggers as possible, and that may require you to throw away or give away tempting foods.

# reality check

**If you are thinking:** *I don't want to throw away food. It's a waste of money.*

**Face reality:** The money is already gone. It's better to waste the food in the trash than in your body.

**Don't be like the dieter who got rid of the tempting cake and candy in her house by eating it! Use this mantra: When in doubt, throw it out!**

If you honestly can't get rid of some foods that might trigger you to overeat, then at least make it as difficult as possible to get to those temptations. Store them in the basement, garage, or even in the trunk of a family member's car. Place them in a closed box at the back of the highest kitchen shelf. Put perishable foods in a paper bag, staple shut the bag, and then move it to the back of the refrigerator or freezer. The general principle is: Out of sight, out of mind.

# task 6

### Make a Memory Box

You will soon start collecting memories of diet-related experiences that are particularly meaningful to you—experiences that have a positive emotional charge. For example, the first time you feel triumphant because you successfully rode out a craving, you'll write down this accomplishment on an index card and insert it into your Memory Box. Keep some blank cards in the box so they will be at hand when positive experiences occur. Or if you prefer, keep a Memory List at the back of your Diet Notebook.

As you progress through Stage 1 and beyond, be on the lookout for these positive experiences:

- When you get a compliment that is important to you

- When you feel really good about mastering a skill (for example, once you make yourself eat everything sitting down for several days in a row)

- When you are so glad you resisted eating unplanned food

- When you suddenly notice that you are rarely experiencing cravings

- When you feel proud of yourself for getting right back on track after making a mistake

- When you realize you are not worried that others are judging you because of your weight

- When you are happy about an improvement in your health due to weight loss

- When you notice how much easier it is to perform a physical task

- When you stay in control of your eating at a restaurant or social event

- When you get through a weekend without overeating

- When you go shopping and fit into a smaller size

- When you get on the scale and see a number you haven't seen in a long time

When you write down an accomplishment, such as sticking to your plan when you were particularly stressed, record how you accomplished this feat so you can use that information again when you encounter similar situations. Storing these memories in your Memory Box or Diet Notebook allows you to vividly recall them when you lose confidence, get discouraged, feel deprived, or think that it's just not worth it to stay on your diet. When you feel as if dieting is too hard, you can pull out your Memory Box and remind yourself why dieting *is* worth it—and that you really can do it!

**tip:** Ask your Diet Buddy to point out experiences that are worth preserving in your Memory Box and to remind you to read your Memory Cards periodically.

# task 7

### Fill Your Distractions Box

In Stage 1, you will learn many techniques to help you follow your plan despite temptation. Distracting yourself—by focusing on another activity—is one such strategy. But the distractions you choose need to be compelling to successfully draw your attention away from food.

In your Diet Notebook, I'd like you to start writing a list of highly distracting activities under the heading "Distractions List." From the list on page 40, choose whichever activities you think would be effective. Keep adding to the list over time as you think of new distractions. Store a copy of your Distractions List—along with any other items you need, such as puzzles, nail polish, playing cards, CDs, photo albums, and the like—in your Distractions Box. Also keep other helpful lists in there, such as friends you can call, Web sites you would like to visit, items you want to buy, chores you never seem to get to, and games you want to learn. Make it as easy as possible to distract yourself when temptation strikes. Consider making one box for home and another for work. You will note that I haven't included reading or watching TV on this list. Many dieters find that these two activities just aren't distracting enough; if they are for you, include them on your list.

## Suggested Distractions List

Read your list of reasons to lose weight.

Read Response Cards.

Read this book.

Read other diet books.

Look up diet Web sites.

Read online diet community support group postings.

Look up low-calorie recipes.

Phone your Diet Buddy.

Do deep breathing.

Play a computer game.

Go window-shopping.

Read magazines in your local library.

Listen to a relaxation tape.

Practice a musical instrument.

Do a jigsaw puzzle.

Do a crossword puzzle from the daily newspaper.

Make or add to a scrapbook.

Organize a closet or cabinet.

Clean out your drawers.

Go to the gym.

Leaf through a catalog.

Talk to a neighbor or coworker.

Play with a child or pet.

Tinker with the car.

Play solitaire or another card game.

Brush your teeth.

Polish your nails.

Call a friend or family member.

Take a walk.

Ride a bike.

Go online and order a birthday or holiday present.

Surf the Internet.

Write e-mails.

Put photographs in an album.

Take a bath or shower.

Do a home-improvement project.

Do a crafts project.

Work in the garden.

Make a homemade or computer-generated greeting card.

Download music.

Brush your pet.

Plan a (real or fantasy) trip.

Read a story to your kids.

Oil the squeaky hinges in your house.

Download some software.

Go to a store and browse.

Take a bike ride.

Drink a low-calorie beverage.

# task 8
## Talk to Your Family

Most dieters don't want family members to mention their eating at all. They don't want to feel as if the "food police" are looking over their shoulders. In fact, many dieters eat quite modestly in front of others because they don't want to be judged— but then they can end up eating hundreds (or even thousands) of calories more when they're alone. It's important to let close family members know that you will be changing your eating habits and are enlisting their support. You don't have to use the word *diet*. You can just tell them that you have decided to eat in a healthier way.

- **Explain that you are reorganizing the kitchen:** "You can help me so much by keeping certain foods out of the house or out of sight."

- **Be nicely assertive:** "I'm starting a new eating program, and I don't want to feel self-conscious, so please don't comment on anything I eat or don't eat."

If some family members are skeptical about your ability to change, shrug it off. They just don't know (unless you choose to tell them) why this time will be different.

# task 9
## Build a Sense of Entitlement

To succeed at lasting weight loss, you have to put yourself first. If you don't, you will have a hard time asking for support, turning down offers to eat, and continually making diet and exercise a high priority. Other responsibilities and activities will always get in the way of your best efforts.

For example, Tina (the names of all dieters in this book have been changed) already had a hectic life. She didn't know how she was going to add diet and exercise activities to her already overly busy schedule. When we examined a typical day, it became apparent that Tina continually put herself last. "I have to drive the kids to school. They don't like taking the bus," she told me. "My husband doesn't like to eat the same foods as my kids, so I have to cook two dinners. I have to drive my daughter to her friends' houses. I have to go to all my son's soccer games." Tina resisted the suggestion to have her family make any changes. "Why should they have to sacrifice just because *I* want to lose weight?"

I was honest with Tina. I told her that dieters who refuse to make time for themselves inevitably fail. I asked her to consider the kind of role model she was presenting to her children. Did she want her daughter to grow up with the notion that she wasn't entitled to take care of her own needs? Did she want her son to grow up expecting his wife to always put him first, even at her own expense? She saw the point. Then I asked her to consider how much of a catastrophe it would be to make some changes. She realized that her family might be disappointed once she stopped catering to their every whim, but they would get over it—and pretty soon her new way of doing things would become the status quo.

Next, we discussed which activities were truly essential, which she could eliminate for now, and which she could delegate to her family. Now, when Tina's schedule gets busy, she figures out what she needs to do for herself first before she schedules other activities. She feels entitled—that she has a right—to do what she needs to do.

Your mindset needs to be, *If my life becomes busy, I still have to put my diet and exercise activities first ... If other people make demands of me, I'm entitled to do what I need to do for myself first ... It's the only way I'm going to lose weight.*

# task 10
## Make Response Cards

Throughout every stage of the Beck Diet for Life Program, you will be creating Response Cards—3 x 5 cards with important messages you need to remember. They are one of the cornerstones of this program, and you will read them every day.

Below are three sabotaging thoughts that most dieters have. I would like you to create the corresponding Response Cards so that you will have them on hand once you start Phase 1.

# sabotaging thought:

### *Dieting should be easy and short term.*

It's no wonder people have such crazy ideas about weight loss. Magazine articles, TV segments, books, Web sites, commercials, and advertisements continually tell you that you can lose weight quickly and without much effort. Well, they are partially correct: If you want to crash-diet and lose *some* weight in just a few days or weeks, you can. *But you won't keep it off.* As soon as you begin to eat more calories, you will start to gain back weight. *It's a biological certainty.*

Here's the truth: Dieting is usually pretty easy at first, when you are highly motivated and see your weight going down fairly quickly. But then it gets harder. And this is true for *everyone.* Unless you have learned the thinking and behavioral skills you need, you are likely to give up when dieting becomes more difficult because you won't know how to motivate yourself to push through. There's good news, though: Hard times always pass, and as you keep practicing and mastering skills, dieting gets *easier and easier and easier.* True, from time to time, dieting will temporarily become more challenging, but every time you push through, it will get easier again.

Achieving success at dieting is just like achieving success in other aspects of your life. You may have to face challenges and overcome obstacles if your goal is to advance in your career, keep a presentable home, maintain your good health, enrich your marriage, or raise healthy children. But the rewards are so great.

To continue to remind yourself of these important concepts, create the following Response Card:

> The only way to lose weight permanently is to learn dieting skills and practice them every day. Then dieting will get easier and easier.

## sabotaging thought:

*This is too much work; I don't feel like learning all of these skills. I don't feel like following my eating plan.*

Many dieters have a rebellious side that can seriously impede their ability to lose weight permanently. If they leave this kind of sabotaging thought unchallenged, they are certain to fail in their long-term weight-loss efforts. They may be able to lose *some* weight, but they won't be able to keep it off. The skills in this program are essential—not optional—for permanent weight loss.

When dieters express this sabotaging thought, I ask them what their goal is. Is it to do what they feel like doing? Or is it to lose weight for good? These two goals are *not* compatible. Dieters can't have it both ways. Since they always say their goal is to lose weight, I ask them to reflect on their past dieting experiences. Has *not* learning these skills led to lasting weight loss? Unless they change their approach, is there some reason that makes dieters think this time will be different?

I frequently give dieters the following analogy: If you had strep throat, would you take only half of each pill the doctor prescribed? Of course not. You'd know that half a pill wouldn't work well enough. It's the same with dieting skills. Picking and choosing what you feel like doing just won't work. You need the full dose. You have to practice *all* of your skills over and over until they become automatic. At that point, dieting will become so much easier. It will require so much less time and effort.

Struggling over whether or not to make yourself practice the skills can be exhausting. You need to put the decision in the NO CHOICE category. Essentially you make the choice not to give yourself a choice. You decide to commit to the program wholeheartedly and to practice the skills whether or not you *feel* like doing them. You decide to follow your eating plan at every meal and at every snack, whether or not you *feel* like doing so.

You have already put lots of other tasks in a NO CHOICE category—at least, I hope you have. I hope you don't struggle over whether to brush your teeth, wear a seat belt, and stop at traffic lights. I hope it is irrelevant to you whether or not you *feel* like doing these things; you do them no matter what. Now, you have to add practicing your diet skills and following your eating plan to this category—*if* you want to be successful in losing excess weight permanently.

Once you accept that you need to practice every skill each day, and follow your eating plan (every meal and every snack) each day, you end the struggle and you increase the odds exponentially that you will lose excess weight and keep it off forever. Make this card:

> I'm choosing to say NO CHOICE. If I want to lose weight, I have to do what I *need* to do, not what I *feel* like doing.

**If I compare myself with non-dieters or maintainers, I'll feel resentful. If I compare myself with successful dieters and maintainers, I'll feel better and be more successful myself.**

## sabotaging thought:

*It isn't fair. Other people eat whatever they want.*

You may know a few thin people who *seem* to be able to eat whatever they want, whenever they want. I wish I could wave a magic wand and grant you the ability to eat whatever you want and still lose weight. But to lose weight permanently, you will have to limit your portions forever. The moment you start eating too many calories is the moment you start gaining weight. But you're not alone in this! It's true for every dieter and maintainer—myself included.

Most thin people *don't* eat whatever they want. *Most thin people are careful.* They continually restrict their eating.

Barbara recently told me that she felt jealous of her sister-in-law, Lauren, because Lauren didn't have to diet. I asked Barbara to pay attention to what Lauren ate. Barbara observed her for several weeks. She discovered that Lauren often left food on her plate. She ate dessert only infrequently and, even then, had just a few bites. At restaurants, Lauren ordered only a main course and often ate half the portions she was served. Barbara later asked Lauren why she ate that way. It was a revelation to Barbara to learn that her sister-in-law consciously limited her eating to avoid gaining weight.

In reality, most people restrict their eating to some degree. When I give workshops on dieting to professionals, I often ask the audience members to stand up. I question, "How many of you eat whatever you want, whenever you want, in whatever quantity you want?" I ask those that do to remain standing and everyone else to sit down. In response, about three-quarters of the audience sits. Then I say, "Would any of you eat more red meat, fried foods, chips, ice cream, pizza, or sweets if there were no negative consequences—for your weight or health? If so, please sit down." Almost everyone else sits down at that point. In audiences of nearly 150 people, it turns out that only one or two people actually eat whatever they want, whenever they want, in whatever quantities they want.

*I* continually restrict *my* eating because I prefer being thinner. I follow the eating program in this book. I usually skip hors d'oeuvres and dessert. I eat smaller portions than I would like. I purposely select foods that are low in calories and high in nutrition. At most, I allow myself one treat a day. I do all this, even though I would rather eat chocolate all day.

If you compare yourself with people who eat more than you do, you will feel continually resentful and deprived. You will experience a sense of unfairness that will sap your motivation. Instead, *you need to compare yourself with people who are successfully dieting and maintaining.* You can be sure *they* are restricting their eating, too.

Please make the following Response Card to address this issue:

> When dieting seems unfair, remind myself that I'm not alone. This is how all successful dieters and maintainers eat. I have a choice. I can let a sense of unfairness overwhelm me, cheat on my diet, and gain weight. Or I can accept that this is what I have to do if I want all of the benefits of permanent weight loss.

\* \* \* \* \* \* \* \* \* \* \* \* \*

Now, with your supplies and Response Cards in hand, you're ready for Stage 1. You're ready to learn the step-by-step skills that will help you stick to the Think Thin Eating Plan—for life. Research from Boston College shows that the people who are the most successful at making any major life change—quitting smoking, giving up alcohol, losing weight—generally start with *one* small step. The confidence they gain from successfully taking that first step leads to the next step … and the next … and the next.

You are about to take *your* first step … and then your second … and then your third … and so on, until you grow into a confident dieter who can stick to the Think Thin Eating Plan in any situation, during any mood, and even when cravings, stress, or negative emotions increase your desire to eat. Let's get you started learning the skills that will not only help you lose weight now and for a few weeks or months, but continually, until you reach maintenance—and then for life.

## Why Other Eating Plans Don't Work

Most eating plans have one or more of the following characteristics. No wonder dieters aren't successful in either losing weight or in keeping it off!

• **Calorie counts are too low.** We have found that most dieters can't sustain an eating plan with fewer than 1,600 calories, day in and day out. They may be able to eat 1,000 or 1,200 calories for a few days, weeks, even months, but they gradually (usually without realizing it) drift up to eating at least 1,600 calories. Or they go above their low calorie count one day, get hopeless or frustrated, and eat hundreds or thousands of extra calories. Then it is very difficult for them to get back on track, and sometimes they eat out of control for days, weeks, or months. There is no point in eating a very restrictive level of calories if you are highly likely to start eating more—you will just gain back weight.

• **Nutritious foods, such as vegetables and whole grains, may be included, but the eating plan doesn't prescribe enough protein and healthy fats.** Foods that contain protein and healthy fats help minimize hunger. But if you spend too many calories on simple carbohydrates, you will get too hungry.

• **Some foods are completely off-limits.** It is unreasonable to think that you won't be able to eat your favorite foods. You just need to learn how to eat them in reasonable portions. Eating plans that say, "You can't eat this ...," or "You can't eat that ...," invariably lead dieters to get off track when they inevitably return to the foods they love.

# Part 2

# chapter 4

# Stage 1

## The Success Skills Plan

Okay, ready to roll up your sleeves? You have reached the part of the program that teaches you the skills you need to get ready for dieting. I can guarantee that either you have never learned all of these skills or you have never been able to consistently use them. That is a major reason you haven't yet been successful. These skills can help you overcome the obstacles that have plagued you in the past. By learning, practicing, and mastering the Success Skills, you will set the stage not only for weight loss, but also for keeping off excess weight permanently. You will learn how to:

**Skill 1:** Motivate yourself daily (page 52).

**Skill 2:** Weigh yourself daily (page 56).

**Skill 3:** Eat slowly, while sitting down and enjoying every bite (page 61).

**Skill 4:** Give yourself credit (page 66).

**Skill 5:** Get moving (page 69).

**Skill 6:** Overcome hunger, cravings, and emotional eating (page 72).

**Skill 7:** Plan and monitor your eating (page 89).

**Skill 8:** Follow your plan, no matter what (page 95).

**Skill 9:** Get back on track—right away (page 102).

Here are guidelines for acquiring these skills:

- **Learn and practice these skills at a rate that feels comfortable to you.** Don't go too quickly! Dieters progress at different speeds. For example, eating everything sitting down is quite easy for people who already have this habit. Others may need to spend days (or longer) mastering this skill. Most dieters need to practice coping with hunger, cravings, and emotional eating many times before they get really good at managing them. But remember: No matter what the skill is, the more you practice it, the easier it gets!

- **Fill out the Stage 1 Success Skills Sheet (pages 266–267) every night.** Don't progress to Stage 2 until you have checked every box for seven consecutive nights. It's important that you master these skills before you start following the Think Thin Initial Eating Plan. Keep in mind that not mastering them never helped you lose weight and keep it off in the past.

- **Contact your Diet Buddy each night after you have filled out the Success Skills Sheet.** You don't necessarily have to make voice contact. You can e-mail or leave your buddy a voice-mail message. Before you talk about anything else, make sure to report on how your weight changed and on which skills you followed and which you didn't. If you weren't able to complete a task fully, ask for help so that you can do better the next day.

- **Try to choose healthy foods and eat reasonable portions,** but remember that you won't put much emphasis on your food choices until Stage 2. Instead, you will focus primarily on building skills now. If you would like to get a jump start, you can do the following:

  - Limit junk food to once a day.

  - Eliminate caloric beverages.

  - Eat vegetables and/or salad at the beginning of each lunch and dinner.

  - Include protein-rich foods at every meal.

  - Eat fruit or protein at the beginning of (or for) each snack.

- **Avoid the temptation to load up on your favorite foods now.** You might have the sabotaging thought, *I might as well eat as much as I want because I'll never get to do it again.* But luckily that's not true! The Think Thin Eating Plan allows you to eat your favorite foods—whatever you want—in reasonable portions, as often as once a day, every day, for the rest of your life. You will learn to plan in advance when you are going to have one, as well as how to limit yourself to a single serving. Think about it: Is it really worth gaining extra weight now? You will just have more to lose when you get to Stage 2.

**Mastering the Success Skills *before* you change what you eat will make the difference** between starting and abandoning another diet—or losing weight for life.

## reality check

**If you are thinking:** *I have to lose weight as quickly as possible. It's okay to change my eating and learn these skills as I go along.*

**Face reality:** The only way to lose weight permanently is to master these skills *before* you start the diet.

# Success Skill 1

### Motivate Yourself Daily

For many years, researchers at Brown University and elsewhere have been gathering records from people who have lost an average of 70 pounds and kept it off for an average of 6.5 years. They created the National Weight Control Registry, which now includes data from thousands of successful maintainers. Many of them had tried to lose weight a number of times before they finally reached their goal and stayed there. What made the difference? What helped them finally achieve lasting weight loss?

These successful maintainers consistently told researchers that their final weight-loss attempt was different because they had more powerful incentives to lose weight and never forgot what they were. The incentives varied from dieter to dieter, but most centered on a health problem ("I want to lose weight to avoid a heart attack") or a social problem ("I'm recently divorced and want to feel confident about dating again"). They never lost sight of those reasons, even after they had reached their goals.

I reached the same conclusion in working with dieters. To be successful, dieters need to motivate themselves continuously. They do so by regularly reminding themselves of the reasons that weight loss is so important to them.

If you're like Emily, a dieter I counseled, you're thinking, *Why do I have to remind myself why I want to lose weight? I'll always remember.* Emily didn't realize that it's really hard to focus on those reasons when it's 4 p.m. and you see those homemade chocolate chip cookies on the breakroom table or it's 9 p.m. and you're dying for the ice cream that's in the freezer. Emily had lots of sabotaging thoughts that pushed the reasons she wanted to lose weight out of her mind in the face of immediate temptation. Do any of the following thoughts sound familiar?

- *It's okay if I eat this.*

- *It won't really matter.*

- *I'll make up for it later.*

- *I've been so good all day.*

- *Everyone else is eating it.*

- *It's too hard to resist.*

- *I'll just have this little bit.*

How many times in the past have you given in to temptation because of thoughts like these? That's why you need a written list of compelling reasons to lose weight and why you need to rehearse these reasons continually—so it's always fresh in your mind why it's worth it not to eat the chocolate chip cookies or the ice cream.

Now, write down your reasons in your Diet Notebook under the heading "Advantages of Losing Weight." Keep adding to the list as weeks and months go by. Emily added many more advantages to her list on page 54 as time went on. Here are just a few:

- I can walk around the lake without huffing and puffing.

- I can cross my legs easily.

- I'm not nervous about losing control of my eating on vacations.

- I hardly ever have cravings, and when I do, I know how to handle them.

- I'm proud of myself every day.

After you make your list, get out the business-sized cards that you bought and write or type one advantage on each card. Now you have an Advantages Deck.

## Emily's Advantages List

Start thinking about all of the reasons you want to lose weight. Most dieters can easily come up with 15 to 20 reasons. Here are the reasons one dieter, Emily, put on her initial list:

- I'll look better.

- I'll feel better about myself.

- I'll have more self-confidence.

- I'll be healthier.

- I'll have more energy.

- I won't have to worry about diabetes.

- My blood pressure will come down.

- My back and knees won't hurt.

- I'll be happy when I get on the scale.

- I won't feel self-conscious all the time.

- It will be easier to go up steps.

- I'll be able to climb the bleachers at my son's games.

- I'll wear more fashionable clothes.

- I'll have a stable wardrobe.

- I won't be embarrassed when I check out at the supermarket.

- I'll be a good role model for my kids.

- I won't feel inhibited when I'm intimate with my husband.

- I'll feel in control of myself and my eating.

- I'll be proud of myself.

- I'll enjoy going shopping.

- I'll feel more confident socially.

- My mother will stop nagging me.

- I'll be able to go hiking with my family.

## When to Read Your Advantages Deck

Along with your Response Cards, read your deck each morning before breakfast to create a helpful mindset for the day. As you read each card (either silently or aloud), be careful not to let the words just pass in front of your eyes. Think about how important each advantage is to you. *Also think about whether you want to go through the rest of your life not achieving each advantage.* It's important to actually read the deck and not just mentally recall what the advantages are. I've found that reading and reflecting on each reason seems to penetrate the mind much more deeply.

Until it's a firm habit, many dieters need a reminder system to cue them to read their decks. The dieters I work with keep their decks in various places: on the bedside table, in the bathroom, on the kitchen counter next to the coffeemaker. Some dieters put them away in drawers but create a visual reminder for themselves. For example, a dieter may put a sticker or sticky note on the bathroom mirror, on the refrigerator, or on a kitchen cabinet. Some dieters like to write "30 seconds" on the note to remind themselves that it doesn't take long to read their decks. Isn't it worth this quick investment every morning if it means you get to lose weight and keep it off?

As you face the challenge of learning more Stage 1 Success Skills and begin changing what you eat in Stage 2, you will find that reading your Response Cards and Advantages Deck once in the morning is probably not enough. You will need to pull them out during the day and in the evenings to motivate yourself to do tasks you may not feel like doing. Carry duplicate sets of your Response Cards and Advantages Deck around with you—in your pocket or purse—so you always have these key motivational tools at hand.

## How to Get Yourself to Read the Advantages Deck

Even though it takes so little time, some dieters resist reading their Response Cards and Advantages Deck. For example, John had sabotaging thoughts: *It's not worth the trouble to read them … I'm motivated to diet now … I'll start reading them later if my motivation goes down.* I asked John if he thought it was a good idea for people to wait to learn to drive on the highway until the first time they needed to travel or if it was worth practicing merging and changing lanes beforehand. He understood the point: It's important to prepare yourself in advance for difficult times.

What John also didn't realize is that reading his Response Cards and Advantages Deck—especially when he didn't feel like it—would build his self-discipline. By practicing doing what he *needed* to do to reach his goal, he would eventually be able to more easily do other things he might not feel like doing, such as sticking to his eating plan.

After our discussion, John wrote the following in his Diet Notebook:

| | |
|---|---|
| | I need to start reading my Response Cards and Advantages Deck now to develop new pathways in my mind so I'll know exactly how to respond to my sabotaging thoughts when they pop up. |

Make sure to contact your Diet Buddy to report that you made your Advantages Deck; reviewed your Response Cards from pages 21, 43, 44, and 46; and marked your progress on your Stage 1 Success Skills Sheet (pages 266–267).

## reality check

**If you are thinking:** *I don't feel like doing this task.*

**Face reality:** If you want to lose weight permanently, you will have to learn to do things you don't necessarily feel like doing at the moment. But the payoff is so great!

# Success Skill 2
### Weigh Yourself Daily

I want you to get in the habit of weighing yourself each morning for the rest of your life. You can do serious damage to your diet if you know you won't have to face the music the next morning. You can also become seriously demoralized if you have followed your diet faithfully all week but the one day you weigh yourself the number on the scale goes up, perhaps due to water retention. You might conclude the diet isn't working when, in reality, it's just a normal, temporary gain. Weighing yourself daily will help you avoid these pitfalls.

Research shows that daily weigh-ins are important. A University of Minnesota study of more than 3,000 dieters determined that only the dieters who weighed themselves daily were able to lose weight and keep it off over a year's time. Dieters who weighed less frequently or not at all tended to *gain* weight. And a Brown University study of 314 dieters determined that people who weighed daily were better able to follow their diets, felt less depressed, and were less likely to binge-eat. A separate study of 209 maintainers found that those who weighed daily were 82 percent less likely to regain their weight compared with those who weighed only weekly.

**tip:** If you suspect that a medication is causing you to gain weight or that you suffer from a thyroid abnormality or other medical problem that might block weight loss, discuss the situation with your health-care provider. Although many dieters I have worked with initially suspected a medical problem was keeping them from losing weight, invariably they were eating hundreds and hundreds more calories each day than they realized.

# It is a biological impossibility for your weight to go down every day.

Are you convinced yet? Here is why weighing yourself daily is so important:

- **It is the only way to desensitize you to your weight and reduce feelings of shame.** Remind yourself that the number on the scale is just a number, not a reflection of who you are.

- **You need to prove to yourself that daily fluctuations are normal.** Even if you've been perfect on your diet, *the number on the scale will go up on some days.* Maybe you had hormonal changes, ate late the previous evening, consumed a lot of high-sodium food, retained water, or experienced some other physiological change. If you didn't know that fluctuations are normal, you might become discouraged. Weighing yourself daily lets you see—time after time—that your weight occasionally goes up or stays the same, but that *it comes down again* as long as you follow the Think Thin Eating Plan.

- **You will need an extra incentive at times to stick to the plan.** When you are tempted to eat extra food, you will be able to say to yourself, *No, it's not worth it ... I don't want it to show up on the scale tomorrow.*

- **You need to learn how to use the number on the scale as information,** making sure your weight is generally going in a downhill direction, even though it won't go down every day. The scale will also indicate if you have plateaued for a period of time, letting you make an informed decision whether it's time to alter your eating or exercise program.

## Getting on the Scale

Are you afraid to weigh yourself? Has it been awhile since you stepped on a scale? I want you to start seeing the number on the scale as a measurement to guide your eating behavior. It's certainly not representative of who you are. It's not an indication of your worth as a person. Here's an analogy that may help: If you woke up one day and weren't feeling well, you might take your temperature and use the information to decide what to do. If the thermometer read 98.6 degrees, you'd probably go to work. If it read 102, you'd probably stay home and call your health-care professional. You wouldn't think, *Oh, this is terrible! I can't believe I let the number get so high! I'm such a failure!* No, of course not. You would just use the number on the thermometer as a guide in deciding what to do.

By weighing every day, successful dieters learn how to avoid feeling disappointed, frustrated, or even overly excited when they see what the scale says. They don't view their weight as an indication that they are weak, inadequate, or out of control. They don't see weight losses as reasons to loosen up or celebrate with food. And they don't use weight gains or smaller-than-expected weight losses as reasons to fall off their diets altogether because they are confident that they know what to do to get the number on the scale moving back down again.

# what to do ...

Weigh yourself on a digital scale tomorrow morning. Today, create this Response Card:

> My weight isn't who I am. It isn't a measure of my worth. It's just a number that tells me important information.

Each morning when you first wake up, read this Response Card. Keep it in the bathroom or put a sticker on the scale to remind yourself. Weigh in your pajamas or undressed—just follow the same routine each morning. Look at the number and then hop off the scale. That's it—you're done! Don't weigh again until the next morning. Some dieters get on the scale two or three times (either immediately or throughout the day), hoping the number will go down, which is a sure sign they are giving the scale too much power. Step on the scale once a day—no more.

It's important to start weighing yourself now, even before changing your eating, because it will help keep you in check. Each morning write your weight on your Success Skills Sheet (pages 266–267), along with any change from the previous day. (You will start to graph your weight loss at the end of Stage 2.)

Here's how one dieter, Sandra, recorded her weight on the sheet:

# day 4

**1.** I motivated myself by reading:
- [ ] My Advantages Deck
- [ ] My Response Cards

- [x] **2. I weighed myself just once. Weight/Change in weight: _172.5/down 0.5_**

- [ ] **3.** I ate everything slowly, while sitting down and enjoying every bite.

- [ ] **4.** I gave myself credit throughout the day for every positive eating behavior.

**5.** I got moving by doing:
- [ ] Spontaneous exercise
- [ ] Planned exercise

- [ ] **6.** I identified hunger vs. non-hunger every time I wanted to eat.
- [ ] I tolerated hunger and non-hunger without eating.
- [ ] I recognized that fullness sets in 20 minutes after a meal.
- [ ] I stopped eating when my food was gone.
- [ ] I calmed down before I ate.

# day 5

**1.** I motivated myself by reading:
- [ ] My Advantages Deck
- [ ] My Response Cards

- [x] **2. I weighed myself just once. Weight/Change in weight: _173.5/up 1_**

- [ ] **3.** I ate everything slowly, while sitting down and enjoying every bite.

- [ ] **4.** I gave myself credit throughout the day for every positive eating behavior.

**5.** I got moving by doing:
- [ ] Spontaneous exercise
- [ ] Planned exercise

- [ ] **6.** I identified hunger vs. non-hunger every time I wanted to eat.
- [ ] I tolerated hunger and non-hunger without eating.
- [ ] I recognized that fullness sets in 20 minutes after a meal.
- [ ] I stopped eating when my food was gone.
- [ ] I calmed down before I ate.

# day 6

**1.** I motivated myself by reading:
- [ ] My Advantages Deck
- [ ] My Response Cards

- [x] **2. I weighed myself just once. Weight/Change in weight: _171.5/down 2_**

- [ ] **3.** I ate everything slowly, while sitting down and enjoying every bite.

- [ ] **4.** I gave myself credit throughout the day for every positive eating behavior.

**5.** I got moving by doing:
- [ ] Spontaneous exercise
- [ ] Planned exercise

- [ ] **6.** I identified hunger vs. non-hunger every time I wanted to eat.
- [ ] I tolerated hunger and non-hunger without eating.
- [ ] I recognized that fullness sets in 20 minutes after a meal.
- [ ] I stopped eating when my food was gone.
- [ ] I calmed down before I ate.

# in session with Dr. Beck

I initially had a hard time motivating Sandra to get on the scale because she hadn't weighed herself in years. Here's how our discussion went:

**Sandra:** I'm really afraid of what the scale will show.

**Dr. Beck:** Well, let's say that the number turns out to be even higher than you think it might be. What would be so bad about that?

**Sandra:** Oh, I wouldn't be able to stand it. I'd feel so ashamed.

**Dr. Beck:** Is there someone you feel close to who also has a problem with weight?

**Sandra:** *[nods]* Yes, my sister.

**Dr. Beck:** Do you want her to feel ashamed of her weight?

**Sandra:** No, of course not.

**Dr. Beck:** How do you wish she viewed herself?

**Sandra:** Well, I don't want her to feel bad. I know she tries. It's just really hard for her. I want her to see that she's really a wonderful person. That having a weight problem doesn't say *anything* about her as a person.

**Dr. Beck:** And what's really important about her, then?

**Sandra:** Who she is inside.

**Dr. Beck:** *[pauses to let these ideas sink in]* So, what does your weight say about you?

**Sandra:** *[thinks]* I don't know.

**Dr. Beck:** What would your sister say it means about you?

**Sandra:** She doesn't care. She'd say she loves me no matter what and that I'm a good person. I know she doesn't want me to feel bad about how much I weigh.

**Dr. Beck:** And what do you think is the most likely thing that will happen as we continue to work together?

**Sandra:** That I'll lose weight, and whatever the number is now, I'll be able to make it go down.

**Dr. Beck:** Ready to get on the scale now?

**Sandra:** *[sighs]* I guess so.

Following our discussion, Sandra did get on the scale. It took several weeks, but she finally became desensitized to the number and was able to use it just as information, without judging herself.

# Success Skill 3
## Eat Slowly, While Sitting Down and Enjoying Every Bite

Many dieters I've counseled were astounded by the impact of instituting these three eating habits. Some said it was the first time they had really tasted all of their food. Many lost some weight, without even trying, even though they had not officially started dieting. Although this skill is difficult for some dieters in the beginning, it's so important to remember that the more you practice it, the easier it gets! Study after study bears out the importance of these habits:

- Research conducted at the University of Pennsylvania determined that diners consumed more overall food and calories when they sped up their eating pace and consumed fewer calories when they slowed down.

- Researchers from Georgia State University and other institutions found that most people ate more when they were distracted by watching TV, talking to dining companions, or listening to music.

- A University of Toronto study found that students consumed more pasta if they nibbled while standing rather than while sitting at a table.

- Research on thousands of Japanese office workers showed that fast eaters ate more calories than slow eaters, tended to gain more weight, and were more likely to have insulin resistance (a precursor to diabetes).

Why is eating slowly, while sitting down and enjoying every bite, so effective? I would like you to do the following experiment to see for yourself. Go to the kitchen and get something you like to eat. Cut or separate the food into two equal portions. Then do the following:

1. Eat one portion as quickly as you can, while standing up, as you focus your attention elsewhere.

2. Eat the other portion sitting down, as slowly as possible, with no distractions. Take small bites. Notice the flavor and texture. Chew each bite thoroughly.

Did you enjoy the second portion more? When you eat while distracted and fail to enjoy every bite, you may want to eat more after eating a reasonable portion, simply because you didn't notice what you were eating. In a study completed at the University of Bristol in the United Kingdom, one group ate in silence and focused intensely on the process of eating. When they finished their allotted portion, they lost their desire to have dessert. A second group ate while playing a video game. These participants reported a high desire to continue to eat—a full 10 minutes after finishing the same-sized portion. Eating slowly, while sitting down and enjoying every bite, helps you cut down on the amount you eat. It helps you in several other ways, too:

**You won't feel as deprived.** Once you start limiting your food, you will want to get the most satisfaction from everything that you eat. You will feel so much more satisfied if it takes you longer to finish what is on your plate.

**You will feel full sooner.** Research shows there is a lag in time from when you have consumed enough food to trigger fullness and when you actually feel a sensation of fullness. The more slowly you eat, the more time you have for the fullness signal from your stomach to reach your brain.

**You will enjoy your food more.** When people eat too quickly, they barely taste what they are eating. I wonder if you do that sometimes when you're eating something you think you're not supposed to have. Do you eat it quickly? If so, does a small piece seem satisfying—or do you keep going? When you start changing what you eat in Stage 2, it will be important for you to get as much enjoyment from each bite as you can.

**tip:** The hungrier you are, the *slower* you should eat. Eating quickly—which may be your first instinct—will leave you feeling unsatisfied and still hungry!

**You will feel more visually satisfied.** Satisfaction is not only physiological, but also it's visual and psychological. If you eat half of your food while you are preparing dinner, for example, then you will have only half left to put on the table. You just won't feel as satisfied—even though you would be eating exactly the same total amount of food—as you would have if you had spread out the entire meal in front of you.

**You will have a calmer mindset.** University of New Mexico research on 25 people who took a course in mindful eating determined that they naturally reduced binge-eating episodes and anxiety during eating.

**You will keep yourself more accountable.** Eating everything slowly, while sitting down and enjoying every bite, helps ensure that you are aware of *everything* you eat. People can consume hundreds (or even thousands) of calories while standing in front of the refrigerator or kitchen cabinet. Many dieters have the sabotaging thought, *Calories don't count if I eat standing up.* But this, of course, is simply not true. *All* calories count. Your body processes calories in the same way whether you eat them while standing or sitting, whether you are fully aware of what you are eating or not, and whether you fully enjoy them or not. So since your body is going to know you ate it, you might as well enjoy it, too!

# what to do ...

It would be wonderful if you could take a pledge, starting right now and for the rest of your life, to eat all of your food slowly, while sitting down and enjoying every bite—100 percent of the time. It's an important goal, one you probably will not reach overnight. It may take you a few days or weeks to master this important skill. *Just keep practicing.* The more you practice, the easier it will get. And remember, it's worth it to make this pledge! You'll get so many benefits in return. Here's what to do:

**1. If you are not already proficient at this skill, you will need reminders.** Put a note that says, "Sit, slow down, enjoy" on the fridge, your kitchen table, and/or your cabinet. Change something in your eating environment: Use different dishes, flatware, napkins, or place mats. If you usually eat in the kitchen, move to the dining room. Every time you notice that something is different, remind yourself: *I'm supposed to eat slowly and enjoy every bite.* Even if you catch yourself in the middle of a meal or snack, it's never too late to use these essential eating habits.

**2. To eat more slowly, put down your utensils** several times during each meal and sip water between bites. Take small bites and be sure to chew thoroughly. You could eat a sandwich in 8 bites—but 20 bites is better. Just imagine how much more enjoyment you would get from 20 bites than from 8. And make sure to swallow each bite before you take the next one. You will find your food and enjoyment last longer.

**3. Make time.** Figure out when you are going to eat each meal and snack, and rearrange your schedule, if necessary. You may need to wake up earlier so you can slowly eat breakfast at home or run errands after work instead of during your lunch break.

**4. In the beginning, eat without distractions.** Try eating alone. Turn off the TV, computer, and phone. Do this for at least three days in a row until you have become accustomed to eating slowly and noticing every bite. It's important to practice this skill even if you have to go out of your way—for example, by eating separately from your family for a few meals. But isn't it worth a few solitary meals if it means a lifetime of weight loss?

**5. Add back in distractions when you're ready.** Try eating while watching TV, talking to a companion, or reading a magazine. See if you can alternate your focus from the food to the distraction and back again. If this task is too hard, go back to eating meals with no distractions and then try again at a later date. Keep practicing—it will get easier.

**6. Figure out how to sit down in each situation—or just don't eat.** If you were on crutches, you would have to find a place to sit, whether you were at a cocktail party, street fair, or supermarket that offered free samples. If there just isn't a place to sit, wrap up the food and take it home. Or skip eating altogether. If your goal is permanent weight loss, you can't afford the luxury of eating while standing. You must break the habit.

**7. Your only exception should be tasting food while cooking.** Take small tastes—and only when you really have to. Eating more than necessary is an unhealthful habit, and it's just not worth spending calories this way. Starting in Stage 2, every bite you eat while cooking is one less bite you will be able to have when you are sitting down eating your meal.

*************

Here are some additional tips I have learned from dieters:

- Allison puts a yellow star-shaped sticky note on the dining table to remind herself to eat slowly. When she finds herself eating too quickly, she stops eating, traces the star with her finger, and slows down. Even when she is out to dinner, she often inconspicuously traces an imaginary star on her place mat to remind herself to slow down.

- Jenna sometimes stops eating and sings to herself when she notices she is eating too fast. She changes the words of Simon and Garfunkel's "59th Street Bridge Song (Feelin' Groovy)" from, *"Slow down, you move too fast …,"* to, *"Slow down, you eat too fast. You want to make this good taste last."*

- Tom makes sure to clear the table completely before he eats. When it's covered with bills, mail, and newspapers, he invariably gets distracted and doesn't enjoy his food as much as he could have.

- Joan delegates cleanup to her husband and kids so she won't be tempted to nibble as she is clearing the table.

Okay, what sabotaging thoughts did you have while reading about this skill? I frequently hear that people think, *I don't want to do that … I don't have time …* or *I don't really need to.…* If, like many dieters, you find that you have any of these thoughts, create a Response Card to read each morning:

> I have to eat every bite slowly, while sitting down, so I can fully enjoy it. It's worth developing this lifetime habit so that I can have a lifetime of being thinner.

It may take some time before you fully master this skill, but keep working at it every day and you will get better and better. In the meantime, remember not to berate yourself—it's not a personal failing. And I promise you *that it will get easier!* If you need help, ask your Diet Buddy. Make sure to contact your buddy tonight to report whether you read your Response Cards and Advantages Deck; weighed yourself; ate everything slowly, while sitting down and enjoying every bite; and filled out the Stage 1 Success Skills Sheet (pages 266–267).

# in session with Dr. Beck

**When I introduced the idea of eating everything slowly, while sitting down and enjoying every bite, Karen was dismayed.**

**Karen:** I'm really rushed in the mornings, and I don't have time to sit down. I just don't think it's that important for me.

**Dr. Beck:** Can you tell me about the last time you ate a lot more than you wish you had?

**Karen:** Hmmm, it was a couple of weekends ago, I guess. It was a Sunday. I was supposed to go to lunch and the movies with my friend, but she cancelled at the last minute. I was kind of at loose ends, and I never really had a proper lunch. I just ate things all afternoon.

**Dr. Beck:** Do you remember what you had?

**Karen:** I picked at some food from the refrigerator at lunchtime. Leftover pizza, I think. Then I ate the last three 100-calorie packs of cookies from the box. I meant to have only one, but somehow I ate all three. I can't remember what I had next. I remember at some point feeling really stuffed and disgusted with myself. I know it just made things worse, but then I ate the last of the chocolate candy from Valentine's Day.

**Dr. Beck:** How much of the food did you eat sitting down?

**Karen:** None of it. I just grazed, standing up.

**Dr. Beck:** Now, thinking back to that Sunday, if you had taken all that food and spread it on the table in front of you and sat down, would you have eaten all of it?

**Karen:** No, I'm sure I wouldn't have. I would have noticed what I was doing. I wouldn't have let myself go that far.

**Dr. Beck:** Exactly. You're exactly right. That's why we've got to make eating slowly, while sitting down and enjoying every bite, such a strong habit—so you can never again let yourself eat on and on.

**Karen:** Okay, I understand. I'll work on it.

**It took Karen several weeks to master this skill. When she did, she was so proud of herself that she made a card for her Memory Box:**

---

Memory Card

I never thought I could do it, but I did! I've gone an entire week eating everything slowly, while sitting down and enjoying every bite. Now I see the point. I really *do* get much more satisfaction every time I eat. And it stops me from mindless grazing and bingeing. Sometimes it's hard to make myself do it, but it's totally worth it.

---

# Success Skill 4

## Give Yourself Credit

Successful dieters continually put the focus on what they are doing right. They tell themselves, *Good job* (or the equivalent), whenever they practice a Success Skill and stick to their eating plan. Doing so builds their self-confidence. They prove to themselves that they really *can* take control and exert self-discipline. In a study at the University of Pittsburgh, participants lost more weight if they practiced skills that increased their confidence, compared with participants who did not take these steps.

Unsuccessful dieters focus too much on their mistakes, viewing themselves as weak, bad, or hopeless. They tend to ignore their small daily successes and therefore don't gain a sense of self-efficacy—a belief that they can, through their own efforts, reach their goals. They get easily discouraged and are more likely to give up when dieting becomes more difficult.

Steve, a dieter I counseled, had this problem. He had worked hard all day to eat everything slowly, while sitting down and enjoying every bite. But he didn't give himself credit. After dinner, he mindlessly ate a slice of orange as he was clearing the table. He focused on this *one* time he had slipped, becoming highly self-critical. Instead of building his self-confidence (he had, after all, eaten his previous meals and snacks perfectly), he eroded it.

## Yes, You *Do* Deserve Credit

Some dieters struggle with the notion of praising themselves. They say, *I don't deserve credit for eating slowly … I should already have been doing that … I shouldn't give myself credit for reading my Response Cards— that should be easy … I should only give myself credit if I lose all of the weight I need to.*

Janet told me that she gave herself credit but quickly negated it every time with the words *yes* and *but.* She would tell herself, *Yes, it's good that I sat down to eat, but it shouldn't have been such a struggle,* and, *Yes, I ate dinner sitting down, but I forgot and popped some carrots into my mouth as I was making the salad.* Janet had the unrealistic expectation that she should be able to master all of the Success Skills overnight. She didn't realize that *everyone* struggles with them to varying degrees.

**tip:** Buy a small counter, the kind people use to keep track of how much their groceries cost while they are shopping or golfers use to keep track of their strokes. Click it every time you deserve credit. Record the number of clicks at the end of the day in your Diet Notebook, under "Daily Credit."

I asked Janet if she had expected her 7-year-old son to read flawlessly in first grade. I had her reflect on what would have happened to his motivation if he had negated his efforts every time he read a page well and criticized himself every time he stumbled. Janet then realized that the perfectionist standards she held for herself were counterproductive, and she began to feel good about her small daily accomplishments.

If you have trouble giving yourself credit, create the following Response Card:

I really *do deserve credit* for breaking old habits, and it is essential for building my confidence. Once my confidence grows, everything will become so much easier.

# what to do ...

**To give yourself credit, do the following:**

**1. Notice every positive eating behavior you engage in**—and every time you refrain from eating something you are not supposed to have.

**2. Say one of the following, or the equivalent, to yourself:** *Good job. Okay! Yes! That was good. Great! Good going! That deserves credit. I did it!*

**3. Write the word** *credit* **on a sticky note.** Place it on the fridge, on your computer, or in your appointment book or PDA to remind yourself to look for times that you deserve credit.

**4. Give yourself credit every time you check off an item** on your Stage 1 Success Skills Sheet (pages 266–267).

Some dieters say it feels unnatural to give themselves credit. Continual practice makes a behavior feel more natural. So try to notice every single thing you do right. Even at this point, before you have finished Stage 1, you deserve credit every time you:

- Read (or reread) this book.
- Read a Response Card.
- Weigh yourself.
- Read your Advantages Deck.
- Arrange your schedule to make time to practice your skills.
- Check off your Success Skills Sheet.
- Contact your Diet Buddy.
- Eat slowly, while sitting down and enjoying every bite.
- Resist engaging in unhelpful behaviors.

Even though we haven't yet discussed how you will change your eating, you can already start giving yourself credit for positive choices, such as when you:

- Serve yourself reasonable portions.
- Refrain from taking second helpings.
- Ignore the baked goods at a meeting.
- Limit your consumption of unhealthy food.

Keep contacting your Diet Buddy daily to report on every Success Skill you are working on so far.

# Success Skill 5

## Get Moving

This program isn't just about losing weight. It's about getting healthy and losing excess weight *for the last time*. That's why it's important for you to start moving *now*, before you have changed your eating habits. The results from the National Weight Control Registry are clear: Nearly all of the successful dieters who have lost at least 30 pounds and kept it off for more than a year exercise regularly. Exercise is important in losing weight and keeping it off for these reasons:

**It helps maintain your metabolism.** Each pound of muscle in your body burns about 35 calories a day as it breaks down and builds up proteins. However, roughly 90 percent of adults are so sedentary that they lose about 5 pounds of muscle mass every decade. Each 5 pounds of lost muscle mass slows total calorie burning (called basal metabolic rate) by about 5 percent. This metabolic slowdown alone can be responsible for a 15-pound weight gain for each decade of life. Dieting without exercise can further slow metabolism. Up to 25 percent of your weight loss may come from muscle instead of fat. You don't want that to happen. Exercise helps reverse this trend, maintaining your muscle mass and, consequently, your metabolism as you lose weight.

**It helps you eat more healthfully.** Regular exercise reduces stress and increases your overall sense of confidence—which can help you combat the desire to eat unplanned meals and snacks. In fact, one of the best things to do when you are craving unplanned food is to go for a walk.

**It helps you control your appetite.** Have you heard that exercise increases appetite? It's true that one isolated bout of exercise can make you hungry as your body attempts to replace the calories you just burned, but research shows that *consistent* exercise normalizes levels of specific fullness hormones, allowing them to more quickly trigger the sensation of fullness when you eat.

**It helps improve your health.** Above all else, this program is about health. Studies show that regular exercise reduces three key factors involved in aging: oxidative stress, psychological stress, and inflammation—which, in turn, reduces the risks for heart disease, diabetes, osteoporosis, and certain cancers. A study at King's College in London of 2,401 twins determined that less physically active men and women—performing fewer than 16 minutes of physical activity a week—were on average biologically 10 years older than their more physically active counterparts (who moved 199 weekly minutes on average), even though they were the same age.

**It helps lift your mood.** Duke University research shows that regularly performing exercise improves mood just as effectively as taking some prescription antidepressants for people who are mildly to moderately depressed.

**It helps you sleep better.** Brazilian researchers determined that physically active seniors slept better and longer than their sedentary counterparts, possibly by helping to regulate body temperature.

# what to do ...

**1. Check with your health-care provider** to be sure that your exercise plan is safe for you.

**2. Start walking a minimum of five minutes every day.** The point is not necessarily to burn calories but to establish a daily lifetime habit of exercise.

**3. If you already do some other form of exercise, keep it up and keep challenging yourself to do a little more.** The American College of Sports Medicine and the Centers for Disease Control recommend that you work up to a minimum of 30 minutes of cardiovascular exercise (such as walking, cycling, or swimming) five days a week, plus strength training two times a week for optimal health. On page 264, you'll find a sample strength-training routine you can do at home. Don't get overwhelmed if you can't initially complete the routine. You can build up to it gradually.

**4. If you don't currently exercise, start some kind of program.** At least three times a week, extend your five-minute walk. Consider going to an exercise class, getting an exercise DVD, going swimming, taking up a sport, doing yoga, or working out at a gym.

**5. Get as much spontaneous exercise as you can.** Walk into the bank rather than using the drive-through. Park as far from the entrance of a building as you can. Take a flight of stairs rather than an escalator or elevator. Do a power walk around your building, inside or out, at lunch. Do a circuit of the mall or supermarket before you start shopping. Every little bit helps.

**6. Make exercise as convenient and enjoyable as possible.** Keep an extra pair of sneakers in the trunk of your car. Change into your gym clothes before you leave work. Pack your gym bag again as soon as you empty it. Ask a friend to walk with you or listen to music or books on CD. Invest in a small TV to put in front of a treadmill or exercise bike.

**tip:** Be careful—don't fool yourself. Some dieters believe they are getting quite a lot of exercise when they shop at a mall or go to a fair because they get tired. Being tired doesn't always mean that you got good exercise. And a 20-minute walk with your dog, who stops at every bush, doesn't give you the same workout as walking fast the whole time.

Andi had myriad sabotaging thoughts about exercise: *I don't want to ... I'll do it later ... It's not worth doing ... It won't help ... I don't need to ... I'm too tired ... I'm not in the mood ... I'm too busy.* Like most people, the hardest part for her was getting started, but once she got going, she was fine. After many misgivings, she finally signed up for a beginners exercise class in her community. When she got back from the first class, she made the following card for her Memory Box (page 38):

---

### Memory Card

I can't believe I was so resistant to sign up for exercise class. It wasn't hard! There were plenty of other people my age there who were just as out of shape as I am. I'm actually so proud I made myself go. I really do feel so much more energized. I'm so glad I did it!

---

After several more classes, Andi was finally able to fully accept the necessity of exercise—not necessarily because it would help her lose a significant amount of weight any time soon, but because it was essential for her well-being, both physically and psychologically. She was finally able to put exercise in her NO CHOICE category.

If you struggle with exercise, reread pages 43–44. Create a Response Card to read each morning and pull it out again whenever sabotaging thoughts threaten to undermine your resolve:

---

Exercise is not negotiable for good health. I need to make it be a daily lifetime habit. The hardest part is getting started. I'll feel so much better when I'm done. So get started!

---

Some people are all-or-nothing exercisers. They think, *If I can't do my whole program, it's not worth doing anything at all.* Others are gung ho at the beginning, but then once they skip a session or two, they abandon their exercise program completely.

If you fall into either of these categories, make yourself another Response Card:

> Remember that five minutes of exercise is better than zero minutes.

When you contact your Diet Buddy tonight—and every night—report on what you did for spontaneous and planned exercise.

# Success Skill 6
## Overcome Hunger, Cravings, and Emotional Eating

You've come to one of the most crucial parts of the Beck Diet for Life Program. I'm going to teach you what to do when you are mightily tempted to eat something you're not supposed to have. If you're like many dieters, you've probably had sabotaging thoughts like these:

- *I'm really hungry ... I need to eat.*

- *I can't resist this craving.*

- *I'm upset ... I have to eat.*

You may have had these thoughts—or variations of them—thousands of times in your life. But I will teach you how to overcome these thoughts so that you can stick to your eating plan.

In the following pages, I'm going to ask you to conduct six experiments that will help you prove the following to yourself.

**Experiment 1:** I often think I'm hungry when I'm not.

**Experiment 2:** Hunger is not an emergency. It's no big deal, and if I get involved in something else, it will go away.

**Experiment 3:** Fullness always sets in within 20 minutes of finishing a healthy meal. I may still feel hungry immediately after I've eaten, but it will soon subside.

**Experiment 4:** I can stop eating when I've finished my planned food.

**Experiment 5:** Cravings are tolerable and go away.

**Experiment 6:** I can tolerate negative emotions without eating in response.

You may not believe these statements now, but you will soon. You will start by proving that true hunger is different from cravings, desire, and other sensations.

# experiment 1

### Prove to yourself that you confuse hunger with other states.

Many dieters label any desire to eat as hunger. But you are only hungry when you experience an empty feeling in your stomach, often accompanied by hunger pangs. If your stomach is comfortable but you feel a desire, yearning, or urge in your mouth, throat, or body, you're not hungry. You are confusing hunger with thirst, cravings, negative emotions, or just a desire to eat. Most of the dieters I've worked with initially thought they knew what hunger was, but they didn't. Whenever they wanted to eat, they thought, *I'm hungry,* even if they had just finished a large meal half an hour before. Labeling their sensations as "hunger" made it feel legitimate for them to eat, even when it wasn't time for them to eat. In reality, many of us want to eat multiple times a day when our stomachs are not empty and we are not experiencing true hunger. It's important to become adept at overcoming this desire so you can control your eating and keep off excess weight for the rest of your life.

True hunger is what you feel when you have fasted for several hours. Your stomach is empty, and you are experiencing hunger pangs. A craving is a physiological and emotionally intense urge to eat. A desire to eat is when you are not particularly hungry, but you just feel like eating. Thirst is marked by a dry feeling in your mouth or throat. When you're upset, stressed, or bored but your stomach isn't empty, you're experiencing a negative emotion—you're not truly hungry.

Once you learn to differentiate between hunger and non-hunger sensations—and what to do when you notice them—you will be better able to stick to your plan. Over time, you may recognize that you tend to desire unplanned food at certain

## What Is That Sensation?

**Hunger =** The gnawing feeling in the pit of your empty stomach

**Non-Hunger =** The desire to eat when your stomach is not empty

times of the month, at certain times of the day (especially when you are tired, bored, or procrastinating), at certain events, when you're feeling negative emotions, or even when you're happy. If you can figure out your triggers, you'll be better prepared to stand firm and stick to your predetermined plan by telling yourself, *No wonder I want to eat … I usually do at this time … But it doesn't matter; I'm definitely not going to eat now … It's worth it to me (and my diet!) to resist.*

# what to do ...

**To learn the difference between hunger and non-hunger, I'd like you do the following:**

**1.** Set up a chart like the one on the opposite page in your Diet Notebook. Label it "Hunger Versus Non-Hunger Chart" and fill it in with your own examples.

**2.** Eat a reasonably hearty breakfast.

**3.** If you snack between breakfast and lunch, skip those snacks (if medically appropriate).

**4.** Delay lunch until you feel hunger pangs in your stomach.

**5.** Every time you feel like eating, fill out the chart in your Diet Notebook.

How will you know whether you are feeling hunger or non-hunger? Notice which sensations you experience in your mouth, throat, and body. Then ask yourself:

- Does my stomach feel empty, and could I feel satisfied if I ate any type of food? (If so, I am probably hungry.)

- Does my stomach feel reasonably comfortable, but I just feel like eating or have a mild yearning to eat? (If so, that's not hunger; it's probably a desire.)

- Does my stomach feel reasonably comfortable, but I have a strong urge to eat a particular food or kind of food, which is accompanied by a sense of tension in my mouth, throat, or body? (If so, that's not hunger; it's probably a craving.)

- Does my stomach feel reasonably comfortable, but I'm feeling tired, sad, bored, frustrated, anxious, or stressed? (If so, that's not hunger; I'm experiencing fatigue or negative emotion.)

- Is my mouth or throat dry? (If so, that's thirst.)

At this point, it's not really important to differentiate between a desire, craving, tiredness or urge to engage in emotional eating, and thirst. You can just label all four states as "non-hunger." For the rest of your life, whenever you want to eat and it's not mealtime or snack time, label your sensations as "hunger" or "non-hunger." Once you master the skill of overcoming hunger, cravings, and emotional eating, you will be able to say to yourself, *This is hunger ... No big deal, I'm scheduled to eat again in a little while,* or, *This isn't hunger ... I'm definitely not going to eat.* In later stages, you will learn what to do to minimize hunger and how to change when or what you eat if you find you are still getting hungry too often.

Here's how Brenda filled in her Hunger Versus Non-Hunger Chart. She ate breakfast at 7 a.m. and lunch at 1:00 p.m. Although there were several times in between when she wanted to eat, she didn't actually experience hunger until 12:10 p.m.

| *Brenda's Hunger Versus Non-Hunger Chart* | | | |
|---|---|---|---|
| Time | Situation | Sensation | Label (hunger or non-hunger) |
| 8:10 a.m. | Packing my son's lunch, want to eat a pretzel. | Desire in mouth | Non-hunger |
| 8:55 a.m. | Walking to work, smell bread baking. | Yearning in mouth | Non-hunger |
| 10:15 a.m. | Feel like procrastinating; thinking about donut in breakroom. | Desire in mouth | Non-hunger |
| 11:20 a.m. | Coworker offers me a pastry. | Urge in throat, body | Non-hunger |
| 12:10 p.m. | At a meeting | Emptiness in stomach | Hunger |

When you contact your Diet Buddy tonight, report on your Success Skills Sheet (pages 266–267) and the conclusions you have drawn from this experiment. Repeat the experiment until it is easy for you to distinguish between hunger and non-hunger.

# experiment 2

## Prove to yourself that hunger isn't an emergency.

If a friend or coworker told you, "I was so busy today that I accidentally skipped lunch," would you think, *Skipped lunch! I can't ever imagine doing that ... I'd get too hungry!*

Many dieters think the same thing. What they don't realize, however, is that hunger isn't a big deal. It just feels like a big deal if you're afraid of it. Many dieters think that they should never be hungry and that feeling hungry is somehow bad or wrong. You may even wonder, *Shouldn't I eat when I'm hungry?* Actually, the answer is, "You should eat only if it's time to eat." It's important for dieters to know that hunger is normal and most people without weight problems get hungry every day, often a little while before meals. If you ask them what they do about it, they usually get a funny look on their faces and say, "What do you mean? I wait for dinner." They know that hunger is not to be feared or avoided and that food actually tastes better when they're hungry.

Most diet programs encourage you to avoid hunger. Some tell you to eat when you feel hungry and to stop eating when you feel full. The problem with that is you are likely to confuse hunger and non-hunger, at least sometimes. Also, since it can take up to 20 minutes for a sense of fullness to kick in, you are likely to overeat at meals because your stomach hasn't had a chance to catch up.

Some diet programs encourage you to fill up on such "free foods" as raw vegetables to avoid hunger. The problem with that advice is that you never learn to tolerate the very normal sensation of hunger. And when free foods aren't easily available, you are likely to fill up on other foods.

Phillip doubted his ability to tolerate hunger, and he engaged in certain unhelpful behaviors to avoid it. He was always thinking about how, when, and where he could get food, in case he got hungry before his next meal. He consistently overate at meals to ensure that he wouldn't feel hungry later on. He kept extra food in various places—his car and office desk—just in case he got hungry. He was continually giving himself the message that it was bad to be hungry, that he couldn't tolerate hunger. This incorrect thinking is exactly what I want to free you from!

People who have never struggled with weight or dieting just don't think too much about hunger. They don't think, *Oh, no, I just finished breakfast ... What if I get too hungry before lunch?* They don't feel panicky during a busy day, thinking, *What if I don't get a chance to eat?* They don't load up on extra food during a meal because they think, *I might get hungry later on.* No, they know that they can tolerate hunger; that it's never an emergency; and that if they turn their attention to something other than their hunger, the sensation goes away. This can happen for you, too, once you overcome your fear of hunger.

Before you start dieting, you need to know, without a doubt, that you can tolerate hunger—because from time to time you *will* feel hungry. The Think Thin Initial Eating Plan will minimize hunger, but it won't eliminate it completely. To avoid ever experiencing hunger, you'd have to eat constantly. Many of the dieters I've worked with have told me that it was such a revelation to learn that they could wait to eat until the next planned meal or snack. Not only were they freed from their fear of hunger, but also they found they actually enjoyed meals and snacks so much more when they were a little hungry.

# what to do ...

**In this experiment, you are going to rate how uncomfortable your hunger really is. Doing so will teach you:**

- You can tolerate hunger.

- Hunger comes and goes.

- You do not have to eat just because you feel hungry. You can wait until your next regularly scheduled meal or snack.

To complete the experiment, you will need to create a Discomfort Scale to rate the level of discomfort you feel during the experiment. Do the following:

**1. Create a chart in your Diet Notebook, like the one Phillip filled out on page 78.** Label it as "Discomfort Chart." You will fill it in with your own examples.

**2. Think back to discomfort you've experienced in your life.** Fill in the top of the Discomfort Chart with experiences in which you felt severe, moderate, and mild discomfort. You will fill in the bottom part when you do a hunger experiment.

## Phillip's Discomfort Chart

| | | |
|---|---|---|
| **SEVERE DISCOMFORT** | | When I had kidney stones |
| **MODERATE DISCOMFORT** | | Last year, when I had that really bad backache |
| **MILD DISCOMFORT** | | Last week, when I had a headache |

| | How much discomfort do I feel right now? | What has been the range of my discomfort during the past hour? |
|---|---|---|
| 12 p.m. | none | none to mild |
| 1 p.m. | mild | none to mild |
| 2 p.m. | none | none |
| 3 p.m. | mild | none to mild |
| 4 p.m. | mild | none to mild |
| 5 p.m. | none | none to mild |

**3. In your Diet Notebook, make a heading called "Hunger Experiment."** Under it, write the following and read this throughout the day you do the hunger experiment:

> Hunger Experiment
>
> It's great that I'm doing this experiment. It will be so wonderful to get over my fear of hunger once and for all. I deserve a lot of credit for doing this.

**4. If your health-care provider approves, tomorrow you will eat breakfast and dinner, but nothing in between.** It's important to know that this experiment is not designed to help you reduce calories for weight loss; it's designed to get you over your fear of hunger. It's fine to drink a little water during the day if you're thirsty. Just don't try to fill up with it, or you will negate the point of the experiment.

**5. Carry your Discomfort Chart with you so that you can make note of any feelings of discomfort throughout the day.** Then every hour on the hour, do the following:

- Rate on your Discomfort Chart how uncomfortable the sensations of hunger are at that moment (none, mild, moderate, or severe).

- Reflect on the preceding hour and record the range of discomfort you experienced.

- Make sure you are rating your discomfort from *stomach* hunger—not cravings, physical pain, anxiety, frustration, or other emotional distress.

- Read your Response Cards.

Are you feeling panicky about this experiment? You are probably more afraid of hunger than you realized. Reflect on a different excessive worry you had in the past—where your fears didn't materialize—to show that just because you predict catastrophe doesn't mean it will necessarily occur. Ever worry about a medical test or loved one who didn't show up when expected? Remember the relief you felt when everything turned out fine? It will be so freeing when you find that your fears about being hungry don't come true and you never have to worry about hunger again. It's a wonderful feeling.

During this experiment, you undoubtedly will feel hungry. You may feel somewhat tired, have a little trouble concentrating, or experience a mild headache. Most people report, however, that the stomach hunger they feel during this experiment is nowhere near as severe as they had imagined.

Phillip was surprised that even his worst hunger was only mildly uncomfortable and certainly tolerable. He was also very surprised to find that even when he was intensely hungry, he didn't stay hungry for a full hour. In fact, his periods of hunger usually lasted about only 10 to 15 minutes and then disappeared. They went away even more quickly when he got distracted.

During the experiment, if you experience substantial discomfort, it's probably not from true physical hunger. Make sure you are rating your hunger discomfort and not your cravings or negative emotions. For example, during the experiment or at other times, you may experience the discomfort of anxiety if you have such sabotaging thoughts as, *Something bad will happen to me if I don't eat.* You may feel tense and frustrated if you think, *I can't believe I can't eat whenever I want to.* It's important to recognize sabotaging thoughts such as these and to respond effectively to them. When you train yourself to think differently about hunger, you will actually feel proud of yourself for experiencing hunger and yet waiting for the next scheduled meal or snack.

You may need to skip lunch on several other days in the coming weeks to convince yourself that hunger is not an emergency. Each time you successfully repeat this experiment, you will become more and more certain that you can tolerate hunger. Keep doing this experiment until you:

- Go from breakfast to dinner without eating and without feeling panicky.

- Change your thinking from *Hunger is bad,* to, *Hunger is not a big deal ... It's only mildly uncomfortable ... I can tolerate it ... It comes and goes.*

Make the following Response Card:

Hunger is never an emergency. It's only mildly
uncomfortable. I can tolerate it. It will come and go.

If this experiment is meaningful to you, file that milestone in your Memory Box. Here's what Phillip wrote on his card:

### Memory Card

I was so afraid of being hungry and so proud of myself
for getting through the experiment. The hunger I experienced was not as severe as I'd imagined. It was actually no big deal. I was amazed.

When you contact your Diet Buddy tonight, report on your Success Skills Sheet (pages 266–267) and the conclusions you have drawn from this experiment.

# experiment 3

## Prove to yourself that fullness kicks in.

If you practice eating slowly, you have a greater chance of feeling full as you finish all of the food on your plate. This sensation won't always happen simultaneously, however. It may take as long as 20 minutes to feel full after eating—which is why it's important to prove to yourself that fullness always sets in, even if it takes a few minutes. Once you know this, when you finish a meal, you will be able to say to yourself, *I'm still a little hungry, but I don't need to eat ... I'll feel full pretty soon, and I'd rather be thinner than keep eating.*

# what to do ...

Make sure you don't have a big snack close to dinnertime so you're at least a little hungry when you sit down. Prepare a good dinner and eat it quickly. Notice how your stomach feels once you have finished. If you don't feel full, set a timer for 20 minutes. Distract yourself with another activity out of the kitchen. When the timer goes off, notice how you feel. Are you still experiencing stomach hunger?

Make yourself a Response Card to read after meals:

> If I feel hungry after a meal, I'll feel full within
> 20 minutes. I don't need to eat more, and
> I always feel so much better when I don't overeat.

When you contact your Diet Buddy tonight, report on your Stage 1 Success Skills Sheet (pages 266–267) and the conclusions you have drawn from this experiment. Continue to set a timer after every meal until you firmly believe that fullness *always* sets in. You may have to do this experiment 10 or 20 times or even more.

# experiment 4

**4** <u>Prove to yourself that you can stop eating.</u>

Now you know hunger is not an emergency and fullness *does* set in. What do you do when you still want more? Many dieters want to keep eating, even though they're not hungry. They enjoy the act of eating and want to prolong it. In this experiment, you'll practice *not* eating—even if tempting food is in front or you—to prove you *can* resist.

# what to do ...

To do the experiment, you will need a Response Card to help you counter the sabotaging thought, *I want to keep eating.* Make a card that says:

> Even though I feel like eating more, it's worth it to me to stop now. I really want all the advantages in my Advantages Deck to come true. Besides, the desire will go away once I get involved in something else.

Then, do the following:

**1.** Plan a distracting activity for after your meal.

**2.** At mealtime, serve yourself a large portion of your favorite food.

**3.** As soon as you sit down, portion off the extra amount.

**4.** Eat the rest.

**5.** Get up and throw away the extra food.

**6.** Note the time and get involved in the activity you planned. See how long the desire to keep eating lasts.

**7.** Give yourself lots of credit for not eating the extra food.

**8.** If this was a meaningful experience, make a card for your Memory Box.

Jason thought he should finish everything on his plate. He was uneasy about eating only some of it. The first time he did this experiment, he wrote this card:

## Memory Card

I gave myself a double portion of meatloaf and mashed potatoes for dinner tonight. When I finished half of it, of course I wanted to keep eating. But I threw away the extra and got busy doing e-mails. I was really surprised. Within a few minutes, I wasn't even thinking of the extra food because I was so involved with what I was doing. I've always been a member of the Clean Plate Club—not anymore!

When I proposed this experiment to Erin, she was horrified—not because it was too hard, but because it violated her rule about never wasting. "Throw away good food? I can't do that!" she said. Erin wanted to wrap up the leftovers, but I explained that I wanted her to get really good at throwing away extra food, a skill she would need whenever food was too tempting to keep. After she mastered the skill, she could go back to saving leftovers. I helped her see that the food would ultimately go to waste, no matter what. To remind herself, she made the following Response Card:

Extra food will always go to waste, either in the trash or in my body.

Tell your Diet Buddy about the conclusions you have drawn from this experiment when you report on your Stage 1 Success Skills Sheet. Repeat this experiment as often as needed until you can easily stop eating and throw away the extra food.

# experiment 5

## Prove that you can make cravings go away.

So far, you have learned that hunger and the desire to eat are not a big deal. They always pass. So do cravings, even though they are usually more emotionally and physiologically intense. The moment you decide you *absolutely will not eat,* cravings diminish. It doesn't work if you are indecisive, though, telling yourself, *I'll try not to have any;* or, *I won't have it now, but maybe I'll have it later;* or, *Let me see how long I can hold out;* or, *It's so unfair that I can't eat this.*

When you experience a craving, your attention gets fixated on food. You try not to think about the consequences of eating it. But it is important to remember that the experience of eating goes far beyond the actual time that food is in your mouth—it includes everything that happens afterward, too: feeling weak, guilty, and out of control (and possibly gaining weight). I would guess that whenever you tried to diet in the past, you gave in to cravings, sooner or later, and felt upset with yourself. Well, you won't have to be at the mercy of cravings anymore, not after you successfully learn how to overcome them by doing this experiment—perhaps many times.

# what to do ...

**1.** Buy a trigger food—a food that you have eaten out of control in the past.

**2.** At home, take out this book and your Response Cards, Advantages Deck, Memory Box (page 38), and Distractions Box (pages 39–40). Pick five activities from the box to try.

**3.** Learn to label what you are experiencing. Create the following Response Card:

> This is just a craving. I don't have to pay attention to it. It will pass.

**4.** Trigger a craving. Unwrap your trigger food, sit with it in front of you, smell it, and imagine eating it until you feel a craving for it.

**5.** Note the time, throw away the food, and leave the room.

**6.** Remind yourself about the importance of strengthening your resistance muscle and weakening your giving-in muscle by rereading pages 19–20.

**7.** Read all of your Response Cards.

**8.** Read your Advantages Deck.

**9.** Imagine the aftermath of giving in. First, think about how disappointed you will be if you give in, the way you probably have many, many times in the past. Then think about how strong and in control you will feel if you resist.

**10.** Try an activity from your Distractions Box. If you finish it and are still experiencing a craving, try another distraction … and then another.

**11.** Once the craving passes, note how much time has elapsed.

**12.** Give yourself enormous credit for doing this experiment.

If this experience was meaningful to you, write a card for your Memory Box. Here is what Sophia wrote:

> ### Memory Card
>
> I can't believe it. I don't actually ever remember actively resisting a craving before. I always gave in! It lasted less than 10 minutes. I don't think I ever quite believed before that cravings go away. They always seemed so intense. Now, I know all the things I can do to wait out a craving.

Sophia, like all of the dieters I counsel, found that this was not a one-time experiment. She needed to do it over, and over, and over again. She actually didn't have to provoke cravings, though—for her, they came on naturally. Once she had a craving, her sabotaging thoughts always started: *I don't think I can resist … It won't really matter if I eat this.* She finally learned that these thoughts were false and that she could indeed resist. She recognized that giving in wasn't worth it because every time

**Think of a craving as an itchy rash. If you scratch it, you will get temporary relief—but the itching will return. If you tell yourself, *It's itchy again ... Oh, well, I'm going to ignore it and keep doing what I'm doing,* it will subside. Turn your attention to something else.**

she did, she strengthened her giving-in muscle, which made it harder to resist (and more likely that she would give in) the next time ... and the next ... and the next. After a while, her resistance muscle became very strong.

Once you get really good at resisting cravings, you should stop trying to distract yourself from them. You should continue reading your Response Cards and Advantages Deck, and just learn to tolerate the discomfort of cravings in the same way that you tolerate other physical or psychological discomfort at times.

Contact your Diet Buddy tonight with your usual report and describe what you learned from this experiment. Whenever you repeat the experiment (through deliberately provoking a craving or experiencing a naturally occurring craving), tell your Diet Buddy about it.

# experiment 6

### Prove that you don't need to eat when you are upset.

Researchers at The Miriam Hospital's Weight Control and Diabetes Research Center in Providence, Rhode Island, determined that emotional eaters were much less likely to lose weight, and much more likely to regain any weight they lost, compared with people who did not turn to food when they felt upset. Luckily, there are many things dieters can do to overcome this problem.

Many emotional eaters feel out of control. Often they feel as if they don't have a choice—they *have* to eat. They just don't know what else to do. Or they feel *entitled* to eat whenever they're distressed, telling themselves, *If I'm upset, I should be able to eat.* But your metabolism doesn't make exceptions. Your body processes calories in the same way, whether you are happy or in distress.

People who have never had a weight problem, as well as successful maintainers, don't rely on food to comfort themselves. The former often don't because it doesn't even occur to them, and the latter don't because they know that they simply can't—not if they want to keep their weight down. Both groups do other things when they are upset. If they have a problem, they try to solve it. They might take some deep breaths, call a friend, or distract themselves. They find ways that don't involve food to deal with their emotions. Or they simply tolerate their negative feelings. You can learn to do the same.

Negative emotions are how your body communicates to you that there is a problem. These feelings are simply a part of life. One reason it's so valuable to overcome emotional eating is that eating doesn't actually solve the problem that has upset you. At most, it serves as a temporary distraction. So as soon as you are finished eating, you will have *two* problems: the original one and also the aftermath of giving in—feeling guilty, weak, and out of control, not to mention gaining weight.

The good news is that emotional eating isn't innate; it's actually a learned behavior, which means that you can learn to overcome it. Once you start working on it, overcoming the urge to eat based on emotions gets easier—and it's so worth it to change.

If for years and years you have used eating as a coping strategy whenever you were upset, you may need to do the following experiment many, many times until your tendency to soothe yourself with food dies away. It's wonderful when you get to the point that you don't even *think* of eating when you're upset. To get there, use every opportunity to repeat the experiment. Initially, you may give in and eat, even after you have used the techniques I suggest. But give yourself credit for any amount of time you are able to resist.

**tip:** Also be on the lookout for overeating in response to *positive* emotions. Julia was very happy when her son announced his engagement. Even though her excitement was positive, she felt physiologically aroused, which was slightly uncomfortable. She turned to food to calm herself down.

Another dieter, Michael, completed a 10-mile bike ride for a charity. He had never done *anything* like that before. He felt elated and proud and, without quite realizing it, raced through the lunch that was provided, hardly noticing what he ate. He then didn't feel satisfied and took seconds— which showed up on the scale the next day.

# what to do ...

**The next time you feel a negative emotion and want to eat in response, do the following:**

**1.** Note the time so you can see how long the urge lasts.

**2.** Label what you're experiencing. Tell yourself, *I'm just upset ... I'm not actually having stomach hunger,* or, *This is just anxiety ... It's not hunger.*

**3.** Stand firm. Tell yourself you're absolutely *not* going to eat and remind yourself why it's worth it not to give in.

**4.** Make a Response Card to help you cope. It might say:

> Emotions are not an emergency. I don't have to eat. I can tolerate this feeling. Eating won't solve this problem. It will only make things worse because then I'll have two problems: the original one, plus feeling weak, guilty, discouraged, and worried that I may have gained weight.

**5.** Take steps to solve the distressing problem, if you can.

**6.** Write about how you feel in a journal, if you wish.

**7.** Talk about the problem with a friend or your Diet Buddy. He/she can help you change your thinking if you are viewing the situation in an unhelpful way.

**8.** Practice techniques to overcome cravings (pages 84–86): Review your Response Cards and Advantages Deck, read about your resistance muscle (pages 19–20), imagine the aftermath of giving in, and try activities from your Distractions Box (pages 39–40).

**9.** When the urge to eat diminishes, see how long it took to go away; write it down in your Diet Notebook so you can remember for next time.

**10.** Give yourself credit for *any* length of time you resisted eating.

The more you practice this skill, the easier and easier it gets, until eventually you won't give in at all anymore. Every time you want to eat for emotional reasons, tell your Diet Buddy during your nightly communication and relate what you did.

# reality check

**If you are thinking:** *I deserve to eat when I'm emotional.*

**Face reality:** If you want to enjoy permanent weight loss, you just can't eat when you're upset. You deserve to feel comfort, but find other ways to achieve it.

# Success Skill 7

## Plan and Monitor Your Eating

I really want you to take the pain out of dieting. The painful part comes when dieters are tempted by foods they know they shouldn't eat and struggle with the decision of whether or not to give in.

James said it was like having an angel on one shoulder and the devil on the other:

*I really want to eat that.*

*—But you're not supposed to have it.*

*But it looks really good.*

*—You know you shouldn't.*

*Maybe I could have just a little piece.*

*—It's not on your eating plan.*

*I know I really should resist, but....*

And then, more often than not, he would end up eating the tempting food.

How many times in your life has that scenario played itself out for you, too? Hundreds? More? It will be so wonderful when you no longer have to engage in this painful struggle.

Planning what you will eat makes it so much easier to resist giving in to temptation. It's very clear: *Here's what I'm supposed to eat, and here's what I'm not going to have.* If dieters want to permanently lose weight, they need to learn to plan their food in advance—and to stick to that plan. In doing so, they will free themselves from the struggle, and once they become very good at it, dieting becomes so much easier. In Stage 4, you will learn how to be more flexible with your eating and will be able to make some decisions about what to eat in the moment. But, first, it's important for you to learn to be an inflexible eater—one who makes a plan and sticks to it absolutely. This is an essential skill that will help you maintain your weight loss for the rest of your life.

Think back to the last time you lost weight and then gained it back. Do you remember how disappointed you were when your weight had gone up? Did you have to return to larger-sized clothing? Why didn't you stop yourself then, get back on track, and lose the few pounds you had regained? The answer is you probably couldn't. It's certainly not your fault—you didn't know *how*. You had never learned the skill of inflexible eating, of making yourself stick to a plan.

Many dieters initially resist this skill. They say planning is just too bothersome or time-consuming. They want to be able to decide what they want to eat when they want to eat it; they simply don't want to plan ahead of time. Dieters tell me that they have lost weight before without planning, so why do they have to plan now? I tell them that it's true—they don't have to plan if they want to lose weight. But if they want to *keep off the weight,* then it's absolutely essential that they master this skill.

And however much dieters protest in the beginning, most actually learn to really like planning. It's a great relief for them to know unquestionably that they can get themselves to eat what they are supposed to and resist what they are not supposed to have. And it turns out to be much easier than most dieters think. In fact, I'd like you to try this quick experiment: Predict how long you think it will take you to write a plan for what you're going to eat tomorrow. Now, time how long it takes to actually write down what you intend to have for all of your meals and snacks tomorrow.

How long did it take? When I do this experiment in my workshops, I find it takes almost everyone between 30 seconds and 2 minutes. I'm guessing that's about how long it took you, too—or at most a little longer. Most people find that there's a big gap between how long they thought it would take and how long it actually *did* take. And dieters come to find out that it is definitely worth spending that minimal amount of time to plan because it helps them lose excess weight and keep it off.

You will continue to practice the skill of inflexible eating until Stage 4. At that point, you will learn the skill of flexible eating and stop writing down a daily plan.

# reality check

**If you are thinking:** *I don't want to restrict my freedom. I want to choose my food in the moment.*

**Face reality:** You will need to give up the freedom of spontaneous eating if you want to reach your goal of permanent weight loss. But isn't it worth it to reach this extremely important goal?

# what to do ...

**1.** Start a fresh page in your Diet Notebook. It should look like this:

FOOD PLAN FOR [date]

|  | Planned | Unplanned |
|---|---|---|
| **Breakfast:** | | |
| **Snack:** | | |
| **Lunch:** | | |
| **Snack:** | | |
| **Dinner:** | | |
| **Snack:** | | |

**2.** Write down what you are going to eat and drink tomorrow. You don't have to write down no-calorie beverages.

Here's what one of Lisa's plans looked like (note that she hadn't yet started to follow the Think Thin Initial Eating Plan):

FOOD PLAN FOR MARCH 21st

|  | Planned | Unplanned |
| --- | --- | --- |
| **Breakfast:** | cereal and milk | |
| | orange juice | |
| | coffee with cream | |
| **Snack:** | pretzels | |
| | yogurt | |
| **Lunch:** | salad with salad dressing | |
| | turkey and cheese sandwich | |
| | pickle | |
| | bag of chips | |
| | iced tea sweetened | |
| |    with sugar | |
| **Snack:** | nuts | |
| **Dinner:** | beer | |
| | vegetable-beef soup | |
| | hamburger on a bun | |
| | French fries with ketchup | |
| | green beans | |
| **Snack:** | ice cream | |
| | microwave popcorn | |

You can see that Lisa had three meals and three snacks. This is what I'd like you to plan, too. Studies show that regularly spaced meals (no more than five hours apart) help you feel satisfied with less food. In a South African study, when men ate small snacks between breakfast and lunch, they consumed 27 percent fewer calories at lunch, compared with when they ate a larger breakfast without between-meal snacks. In Stage 4, you will be able to experiment with eating larger meals and skipping some or all of your snacks.

For now, though, it's important to learn the skill of planning three meals and three snacks a day—and sticking to this plan. At this point, you can plan whichever foods you want, and you don't have to write down quantities. You need to learn this skill of planning your meals in advance so you can fall back on it any time in the future that you put on a few pounds. It will help you gain a sense of control over your eating.

## How to Monitor Your Eating

The next step is to keep track of every bite you eat and every sip of a caloric beverage you drink, even if it's a miniscule amount. Remember, it's not just the calories I'm trying to make you more aware of. I want you to be fully conscious of every time you strengthen your resistance muscle and every time you strengthen your giving-in muscle. It's not only about the calories; it's about the *habit*.

Do the following:

**1.** Carry your Diet Notebook with you throughout the day and check off each food as you eat it. (Don't wait until later in the day to do this.)

**2.** Cross off any food you had planned to eat but didn't consume.

**3.** Write down any unplanned eating.

*Recording all of your unplanned eating is essential because you need to squarely face all of your mistakes* and devise ways to avoid making them in the future. Recording unplanned eating is also important because it can help show you if you are planning your meals and snacks appropriately. For example, if you notice that you often eat unplanned food in the afternoon, you may need to plan more protein at lunch and a more substantial snack between lunch and dinner.

See how Lisa monitored what she ate on page 94. Note that she did not eat the green beans she had planned to have at dinner, and she ate an unplanned cracker in the morning and baby carrots in the afternoon.

When dieters don't write down their unplanned food, chances are very likely they will forget they ate them. University of Chicago research completed on athletes, teenagers, and obese participants showed that nearly all people of all ages, weights, and fitness levels underestimate their food intake—some by as much as 50 percent.

```
FOOD PLAN FOR MARCH 21st

                        Planned                    Unplanned

Breakfast:      ✓cereal and milk
                ✓orange juice
                ✓coffee with cream

Snack:          ✓pretzels
                ✓yogurt                     a cracker

Lunch:          ✓salad with salad dressing
                ✓turkey and cheese sandwich
                ✓pickle
                ✓bag of chips
                ✓iced tea sweetened
                    with sugar

Snack:          ✓nuts                       baby carrots

Dinner:         ✓beer
                ✓vegetable-beef soup
                ✓hamburger on a bun
                ✓French fries with ketchup
                green beans

Snack:          ✓ice cream
                ✓microwave popcorn
```

The study found even thin people forget to account for an average 20 percent of their daily food intake if they merely try to remember what they eat rather than write it down. The dieters I counsel forget about the cream in their coffee, the doughnut at an office meeting, the free cheese sample at the grocery store, the wine before dinner, and so on. And research from Bowling Green State University on 40 dieters determined that those who wrote down their food choices for six months lost nearly twice as much weight as dieters who did not write down what they ate.

# reality check

**If you are thinking:** *I just don't want to do this. I really don't think I have to. I can just plan in my head.*

**Face reality:** If you don't learn this important skill now, you will be at an extremely high risk of not reaching your goal to lose weight for good. Ask yourself, *Which is more important to me? Not planning my food or getting to keep off weight for the rest of my life?*

You will continue writing down your daily eating plan, carrying your Diet Notebook to monitor in writing what you eat, and checking off this skill on your Success Skills Sheet (pages 266–271) until Stage 4. Give a full report to your Diet Buddy every night.

# Success Skill 8

## Follow Your Plan, No Matter What

Don't worry, I'm not going to just tell you to stick to your plan without teaching you *how* to do it. I'm going to provide you with 11 Resistance Techniques so you will know exactly what to do when temptation strikes. You have been practicing many of these techniques since you started working on Success Skill 6: overcoming hunger, cravings, and emotional eating. How do you get good at following your plan? Practice, practice, practice! The more you practice, the easier these techniques will become.

Many dieters are able to do quite well following their plans on weekdays but find it more difficult in the evenings and on weekends. If you do, too, then structuring your time will be a great help. Initially you may want to spend more time than usual out of the house while you are learning this skill.

When Lisa first started planning her meals and snacks, she knew it would be difficult to limit herself to just one evening snack, since she was accustomed to "grazing" until she went to bed. So she made plans to go out every night for a week: She went to the library and read magazines, met her best friend for coffee, window-shopped at the mall, visited her sister, volunteered in the community, and saw movies. At home, she practiced the Resistance Techniques described on the following pages. After a week, Lisa no longer had to routinely leave the house. For the next few weeks, she occasionally left when her control was shaky, but the more she practiced her Resistance Techniques, the more she found she just didn't need to go out.

# what to do ...

Whenever you are tempted to eat unplanned food, use as many Resistance Techniques as necessary. In your Diet Notebook, start a new page with the heading "Resistance Techniques." After you practice them, reorder them according to their effectiveness.

## resistance technique 1

**1** **Say to yourself, *NO CHOICE*.**

This short phrase helps eliminate the struggle involved with following a plan. Make the choice *not* to give yourself a choice about eating unplanned food. (When you get to Stage 4, you will learn how to eat with more flexibility.) Think how much easier life would be if every time you were tempted, you were able to confidently say to yourself, *NO CHOICE. That's it. I'm absolutely not going to eat it!*

Pull out the Response Card you made on page 44 or make one that is simpler:

NO CHOICE

It will be important for you to read this card whenever you feel the struggle to eat unplanned food. Some days you may need to read it quite a few times.

**Once you have made the decision that you're going to follow your plan *no matter what,* you gain a wonderful sense of control.**

......................................................................................................

# resistance technique 2

**Say to yourself, *Oh, well.***

*Oh, well,* is a shorthand way of saying:

> *I don't like this situation but I can't change it, so I may as well stop struggling, accept reality, and move on.*

In the context of dieting, it means:

> *I don't like the fact that I have to restrict my eating right now, but I have to if I want to lose weight and keep it off. I may as well accept this fact, stop the mental struggle, and go find something else to occupy my mind.*

You can add the following idea, too:

> *Besides, although I may not like restricting my eating right now, I will definitely like all of the benefits of losing weight.*

The technique of saying *Oh, well* can be applied to all sorts of situations. When you find that the line at the supermarket is slow, you can get frustrated—or say, *Oh, well.* You can get angry at the inconsiderate driver in front of you—or you can say, *Oh, well.* You can get upset when you have to move an event inside because it has started to rain—or say, *Oh, well.*

If those two words don't grab you, here are some alternate phrases dieters I have counseled have used: *Move on. Let it go. Get over it. Never mind.* Create a Response Card with the saying you like best.

# resistance technique 3

### Dispute your *I don't care* voice.

The tricky part about this sabotaging thought is that it is probably true—in the moment. Fixating on food crowds out your voice of reason. Reread this Response Card from page 21:

> It is true that I don't care at this very moment. But if I eat this unplanned food, I am going to care quite a lot in just a few minutes. I know I will feel really bad if I give in, but I will feel terrific if I resist. I need to go do something else!

# resistance technique 4

### Quell your "adolescent rebellion."

That's what Erica calls the voice that says, *I'm going to do what I want ... I'm going to eat this unplanned food.* It's wonderful to have a childlike part that is lighthearted and free. It's terrible if it keeps you—the adult—from achieving a very important goal or deprives you of the benefits of losing weight. When you think, *I'm not going to follow my plan because I don't want to,* read the following Response Card:

> "I don't want to" is just my adolescent rebellion talking. I'm not going to pay attention to it.

# resistance technique 5

If I'm not supposed to eat something, I will remind myself, *Just because I feel like eating doesn't mean I should … There's no emergency … I'll be so glad in a few minutes if I don't give in.*

Successful dieters and maintainers stay successful because they don't eat whatever they want, whenever they want it. They stick to their plans.

Every time I resist eating something I'm not supposed to have, I strengthen my resistance muscle—which will make it easier and easier and easier to resist in the future.

Every time I eat something I'm not supposed to eat, I strengthen my giving-in muscle—which makes it more likely that I'll give in the next time … and the next … and the next.

If I eat this unplanned food, I'll get momentary pleasure, but then I'll definitely feel bad afterward. It's not worth it!

Either I deprive myself of eating this food today or it's highly likely that I will deprive myself forever of all of the advantages of losing weight.

If I want to lose excess weight forever, I need to stick to my plan—no ifs, ands, or buts.

I can always plan to eat this food tomorrow.

## resistance technique 6

**Drink water or a low-calorie beverage if you're thirsty.**

Water doesn't have any magical weight-loss power, but if you are thirsty and not hungry, it can ward off an urge to eat unplanned food.

## resistance technique 7

**Meditate, pray, or relax.**

Try one of the following breathing techniques:

- Take 10 deep, s-l-o-w breaths in through your nose and out through your mouth. Concentrate on your breathing. If you start to think about food, gently bring your attention back to your breathing.

- Change your breathing, inhaling very shallowly through your nose (so that your chest does not rise) and s-l-o-w-l-y count to four. Then exhale shallowly as you s-l-o-w-l-y count to four. Do this for two to five minutes. If you start to think about food, gently bring your attention back to counting and breathing.

# resistance technique 8

### Read your Advantages Deck.

After you read each card, ask yourself the following questions:

- *How important is this advantage to me?*

- *How important is eating this food to me?*

- *Which would I rather have: this advantage or this food?*

# resistance technique 9

### Do a negative fast-forward.

Imagine, in detail, how you will feel 10 minutes after eating the unplanned food. Visualize the situation: Will you feel weak and out of control? Disappointed with yourself? Nervous about getting back in control? Hopeless about ever losing weight? Discouraged that you have undermined your hard work? Remind yourself how many times you've given in before and how you felt afterward. Ask yourself, *Will eating this unplanned food* really *be worth a few moments of pleasure?*

# resistance technique 10

### Do a positive fast-forward.

Imagine, in detail, how you will feel 10 minutes after resisting the unplanned food. Visualize how you will feel: Strong and in control? Proud of yourself? Hopeful that you will get to your goal? Delighted that you exercised your resistance muscle? See yourself tomorrow morning when you get on the scale. Think about how good you will feel that you didn't give in. Once you see the entire picture, ask yourself, *Which seems better: eating or not eating unplanned food?*

# resistance technique 11

### 11 Distract yourself.

This will help you wait out the urge to eat. Get out the Distractions Box you created in Chapter 3 (pages 39–40). First, start the activity that you think will be most distracting. If you finish it and the urge to eat has not gone away, try a second activity and so on. Remember that watching TV and reading are often not distracting enough (especially if you are used to eating while engaging in these activites); listening to music helps some people but not others.

When you contact your Diet Buddy from now on, report on which techniques helped the most.

**tip:** Do not use chewing gum as a resistance technique. Some dieters tell me, "I can resist tempting foods, but only if I chew a piece of gum." To effectively exercise your resistance muscle, you need to get accustomed to eating three meals and three snacks *with nothing else in between*. It's okay to enjoy an occasional piece of gum, but don't pop it in your mouth because you think, *I need it*. Once you learn to tolerate the sensation of having an empty mouth, you will be truly free.

# Success Skill 9

### Get Back on Track—Right Away

You may not realize that all long-time maintainers, and even people who have never had weight problems, overeat from time to time. Why don't they gain weight? Because they don't think about it catastrophically. Instead, they just use their skills to get back on track immediately. They don't get down on themselves. They don't get hopeless. They tell themselves, *Okay, I wish I hadn't done that … Oh, well, I'll eat a bit less the rest of today.*

Unsuccessful dieters do just the opposite. Instead of immediately getting problem-solving oriented, they lose perspective and then make poor decisions. When they eat something they shouldn't, they often tell themselves, *This is terrible! I'm so weak! I lost control! I can't believe I did that! I might as well give up and eat whatever I want for the rest of the day because, starting tomorrow, I'll have to cut my calories way back and deprive myself.*

It's interesting that dieters can be so rational and reasonable in other areas of their lives. But when they go off their diet, they somehow think it is okay to compound one mistake with another. In fact, it doesn't make sense to eat one unplanned food and then go on to eat much more. Think about it this way: If you got a ticket for running

**Mistakes are not the end of the world,** and they are not the end of your diet—as long as you know how to respond to them. **Successful maintainers make mistakes,** but they recover from them right away.

・・・・・・・・・・・・・・・・・・・・・・・・・・・・・・・・・・・・・・・・・・・・・・・・・・・・・・・・・・・・・・・・・・・・・・・・・・・・・・・・・・・・・・・・・・・・・

a red light, would you continue to run red lights for the rest of the day? Would you say, *I might as well run as many as I want and start again tomorrow?* Of course not! You would stop at the very next red light you encountered.

To lose weight successfully, you need to learn how to stop yourself at the first mistake, put it in perspective, and recommit yourself right away. Because that's just what it is: *a mistake.* We are all human and, therefore, not perfect, so mistakes are an inevitable part of life. I don't know a single dieter who followed a plan perfectly, day in and day out for the rest of his/her life. *I still make mistakes from time to time.* But I limit them and get back on track right away. Expect to make mistakes from time to time and expect to use all of your skills so you can get back on track right away, too.

To help yourself respond quickly to mistakes, I'd like you to use a Cheat Sheet (page 104) every time you eat unplanned food. It will help you view mistakes as learning experiences rather than catastrophes. Instead of feeling guilty and bad about yourself when you make a mistake, you will be able to benefit from the experience. The Cheat Sheet will help you evolve from thinking, *I've blown it … I might as well start over tomorrow,* to thinking, *Big deal, I made one mistake … I deserve a lot of credit for stopping now … This is a good sign that I'll be successful in the future.*

---

### The One Situation in Which You Shouldn't Eat When You Planned To …

It's actually very important to refrain from eating if you are feeling upset, stressed, or rushed—even if it's time to eat. It's important to wait because you can't possibly enjoy your food when you're feeling this way, and you are likely to feel unsatisfied and overeat.

---

# what to do ...

To make your Cheat Sheet, get a 3 x 5 card. On it, write the following questions:

- What was the situation, and what were my sabotaging thoughts?
- Did I eat this food slowly, while sitting down and enjoying every bite?
- How do I feel now that I've given in?
- Had I read my Response Cards and Advantages Deck today?
- Did I try any other Resistance Techniques?
- How can I avoid this situation in the future?
- What can I say to myself next time?

Carry this card with you. Take it to an office-supply store and have it laminated. Whenever you eat unplanned food, pull it out and think about your answers to those questions. For example, when Grace found herself taking a second helping of ice cream one night, she pulled out the card. This is how she answered the questions:

- **What was the situation, and what were my sabotaging thoughts?** I finished eating ice cream. I thought, *That was good ... I really want more ... I just can't resist.*

- **Did I eat this food slowly, while sitting down and enjoying every bite?** No, I ate it standing at the kitchen counter, spooning the ice cream directly from the container. I definitely didn't fully taste it or enjoy it.

- **How do I feel now that I've given in?** Guilty and disappointed.

- **Had I read my Response Cards and Advantages Deck today?** Yes, in the morning.

- **Did I try any other Resistance Techniques?** No.

- **How can I avoid this situation in the future?** I can read my Advantages Deck before having this snack at night to remind myself why it's worth it not to eat more. And then, once I'm finished, I can immediately wash my bowl and spoon, brush my teeth, and get involved in something else. If I'm too tempted next time, I can just throw away the rest of the pint of ice cream. Better wasted in the trash than in my body!

- **What can I say to myself next time?** *It's not worth the few moments of pleasure—it won't be that pleasurable anyway because I'll feel guilty about it and I won't really be able to enjoy it. I'll be really glad if I resist.*

## In choosing to follow this program—in order and as described—you are choosing not only to lose weight, but also to lose weight for life.

Write your Cheat Sheet answers in your Diet Notebook. Read them periodically—even when you don't need them—to keep your answers and helpful problem-solving ideas fresh in your mind.

**tip:** Consider making a Cheat Sheet card for your Diet Buddy, so your buddy can review the questions with you the next time you stray.

### Before You Move On

Master all Stage 1 skills before you move on to Stage 2. If you don't, I predict you will have a hard time—sooner or later—sticking to the Think Thin Initial Eating Plan. Make sure you check off all skills for seven consecutive days before moving on—it doesn't matter how long it takes. And be sure to keep increasing exercise.

You're ready to move on to Stage 2 once you've not only checked off each skill for seven consecutive days, but you *also* firmly believe that:

- If I'm hungry or craving or just want to eat for emotional reasons, it's no big deal. These aren't emergencies. I know what to do to resist. I can wait until my next scheduled meal or snack.

- If I'm tempted to eat something I haven't planned, I have to use Resistance Techniques. It's worth it to me not to give in.

- If I get off track, I need to get back on immediately.

## reality check

**If you are thinking:** *I haven't mastered these Stage 1 skills, but I think I'll move on to changing my eating and work on my skills along the way.*

**Face reality:** It just doesn't work to move on without mastering these skills. If you don't master them now, chances are you never will. Once you start Stage 2, you will be busy with changing your eating. It's likely you will be successful in losing some weight, but you are unlikely to be able to keep it off.

# chapter 5

# Stage 2

## The Think Thin Initial Eating Plan

The Think Thin Eating Plan (which is made up of the Initial Eating Plan and the Lifetime Eating Plan) is a nutritious diet that you can feel comfortable sticking with for life. It features an assortment of meal options, which not only are delicious but also contain optimal amounts of fiber, healthful fats, lean protein, calcium, and other important nutrients. These balanced meals are satisfying and have helped the dieters I counsel to lose excess weight, keep it off, and improve their overall health and well-being in the process. They find that they have fewer cravings. Their blood-sugar levels are more stable. Their moods lift. They have more energy. Many even find that they sleep more soundly at night. You might not realize that a poor diet can negatively affect all of these things, but it really can.

The Think Thin Eating Plan is customized for you. You will determine your initial calorie level on the facing page and find the corresponding formula for what to eat for each meal and snack on pages 210–214. You will use the formula to choose main dishes, side dishes, snacks, condiments, Add-On Calories, and Bonus Calories from lists on pages 215–227. Add-On Calories allow you to add extra ingredients to dishes to make them even more tasty. Bonus Calories are an allotment of 150 or 200 calories that you will spend every day on any food or beverage you'd like. You can create your own meals or use the recipes in Chapter 11. And I've simplified the process by determining portion sizes and doing the calorie counting for you.

As you transition to Stage 2, make it your goal to follow your plan *no matter what*, using Resistance Techniques (pages 96–102) to stay in control. The more you practice these techniques, the better you will get at using them and the less you will struggle. Resisting unplanned food will become easier and easier. When it does, you will be ready to learn how to handle the challenging situations presented in Stage 3 and transition into the Think Thin Lifetime Eating Plan in Stage 4, in which you will learn to eat more flexibly, adjust your plan in the moment, adapt personal recipes, and much more. But at this stage, it's important to learn to continually flex your resistance muscle by following your plan inflexibly, which will help you build the control to make good spontaneous eating choices in the future.

## Determine Your Calorie Level

The Think Thin Eating Plan offers five calorie levels: 2,400; 2,200; 2,000; 1,800; and 1,600. You will start with the highest level that still enables you to lose weight. Once you plateau for a few weeks, you will move down one level. To find the right starting level, use a calculator to compute the math.

| | WOMEN | | MEN |
|---|---|---|---|
| **A** | Your age in years x 7.31 = _519_ | **A** | Your age in years x 9.72 = ____ |
| **B** | 387 – A = ____ | **B** | 864 – A = ____ |
| **C** | Your weight in pounds x 4.95 = ____ | **C** | Your weight in pounds x 6.46 = ____ |
| **D** | Your height in inches x 16.78 = ____ | **D** | Your height in inches x 12.8 = ____ |
| **E** | C + D = ____ | **E** | C + D = ____ |
| **F** | B + E = ____ | **F** | B + E = ____ |
| **G** | F – 200 = ____ (your calorie goal) | **G** | F – 200 = ____ (your calorie goal) |

Adapted with permission from the National Academies Press, Copyright 2005, National Academy of Sciences

Depending on your age, you may get a negative result for Step B. In that case, for Step F, you would simply subtract the smaller (negative) number from the larger number.

For example, here is how a 5'7" 65-year-old woman weighing 195 pounds arrived at her 1,800-calorie level:

**A**  Your age in years x 7.31 = <u>475.15</u>

**B**  387 – A = <u>-88.15</u>

**C**  Your weight in pounds x 4.95 = <u>965.25</u>

**D**  Your height in inches x 16.78 = <u>1124.26</u>

**E**  C + D = <u>2089.51</u>

**F**  B + E = <u>2001.36</u>

**G**  F – 200 = <u>1801.36</u> (your calorie goal)

Regardless of your age, the answer you get in Step G is the number of calories you need to consume to lose weight slowly and steadily, assuming you are currently exercising fewer than 30 minutes a day. (If you are exercising longer, multiply your calorie goal by 1.2.) Round up or down to the closest calorie level. For example, if your answer is 2,150, you will use the 2,200-calorie plan; if your answer is 2,075, you will use the 2,000-calorie plan.

Before you start, make sure your health-care provider approves of the calorie level you calculated on the Think Thin Eating Plan. Keep the following pointers in mind during the first couple of weeks that you are fully on the plan:

- If you don't lose weight within the first week, you are either on a plan that contains too many calories (and you will need to step down to the next level) or you have not followed the plan precisely. Make sure you are counting every ingredient, measuring every portion, and eating your meals at home.

- If you often feel intensely hungry and lose more than 2 pounds during the second and third weeks of this eating approach, you are following a calorie plan that is too low. Step up one level.

- If you start with the 1,600-calorie plan and don't lose weight, do one of the following:

  - Decide to use this plan to help you eat in a healthier way and maintain your weight.

    **OR**

  - Increase your exercise to lose weight (if it's reasonable to do so).

    **OR**

  - Consult a registered dietitian to help you reduce your calories to 1,400 (if you need to lose weight to improve your health).

# in session with Dr. Beck

Carrie was disappointed when I suggested that she start at the 2,200-calorie level.

**Carrie:** But it will take *forever* to lose weight if I eat that much. In the past, I've always been on 1,200-calorie diets.

**Dr. Beck:** Tell me about that. How much have you lost on 1,200 calories?

**Carrie:** I usually lose between 20 and 25 pounds. Once I lost 32 pounds.

**Dr. Beck:** And then what happened?

**Carrie:** Well, I always gained it back.

**Dr. Beck:** Right. Now, one reason you may have gained it back is that you didn't have the skills you needed to stay on the diet long term. But a second reason may very well be that you just can't sustain a 1,200-calorie diet, day in and day out, year after year.

**Carrie:** But doesn't it make sense to start at the 1,200-calorie level and, after I get to my goal, go up then?

**Dr. Beck:** If you lose weight on 1,200 calories and plateau there, you will gain back weight when you start eating more than 1,200 calories. And then you run the risk of getting demoralized and giving up dieting altogether. Is that what happened in the past?

**Carrie:** *[thinks]* Yes, I guess so.

**Dr. Beck:** What I'd like to suggest is that you start at 2,200 calories. Then when you plateau, you'll go down to 2,000, if you still want to lose more.

**Carrie:** I get it, but I'd still like to lose weight more quickly.

**Dr. Beck:** Of course. I wish I could say that it's likely you could lose weight quickly and keep it off. But that has just not been my experience.

**Carrie:** *[sighs]* Okay.

**Dr. Beck:** Think of it this way. You'll lose more slowly, but once you take off the weight, you have an excellent shot at never putting it back on again—if you don't make the mistake of cutting your calories to a level that you just can't sustain. Besides, if it takes a month or a year to lose the weight, does it really matter as long as it will be off for the rest of your life?

**Carrie:** No, I guess not.

Even if you're skeptical about your ability to lose weight at the suggested level, give it a try! I often find that if dieters had trouble losing weight in the past at a specific calorie level, it's very possible that they were actually eating (at least) several hundred extra calories most days through cheating; eyeballing their portions; forgetting some of the food they ate; not counting all ingredients; underestimating the calories they consumed when eating out; or eating and drinking much more on holidays, on weekends, and at special events. Dieters might have followed a certain calorie level faithfully for part of the week but often ate considerably more on other days (especially on the weekends). Like most dieters, you will be happy to see that you can follow a higher-calorie plan than you might think and still lose weight. And you will be much more satisfied and comfortable doing so.

## How to Transition Your Eating

You will continue to plan three meals and three snacks as practiced in Stage 1, but now you will also start choosing foods from the Think Thin options, which you will incorporate at the rate that works best for you. Progress using one of the following three speeds:

**Slow Speed:** Change one meal at a time, starting with breakfast. Once you feel comfortable using the Think Thin Breakfast Options, then add lunch ... then dinner ... then snacks ... and then Bonus Calories (150 or 200 daily calories that you can use for any foods or beverages that you wish).

**Medium Speed:** Change your main meals (breakfast, lunch, and dinner) first. Once you feel comfortable with the options for these meals, change your snacks and add in Bonus Calories. If you choose this speed and find you have difficulty, try moving back to the slow route.

**Fast Speed:** Change all of your meals, snacks, and Bonus Calories at the same time. If you choose this speed and have difficulty, move back to the slow or medium route.

Next, turn to pages 210–214 to find the formula for the calorie level you calculated on page 107. The formula will guide you in choosing specific foods and portions from the lists on pages 215–227. If you are starting at the slow speed, select breakfast foods from these lists and write them down on your Food Plan. Record whichever foods you want for your other meals and snacks. If you are starting at a faster speed, use the corresponding lists for your food selections.

Remember, your ultimate goal is long-term success. I've found that many dieters do better if they slowly ease into the Think Thin Initial Eating Plan. Although they may lose weight more slowly, they are often better able to make permanent changes in their eating—changes that will help them lose weight for life. And, anyway, isn't that why you chose this program? After all, you can lose weight with any diet, but on this one, you can lose excess weight *permanently!*

## Sample Food Plan Chart

Below is how Cindy, who was following the 2,000-calorie level, filled in her Food Plan Chart. Note that she ate 12 almonds she hadn't planned to have and also consumed 1 extra cup of frozen yogurt.

FOOD PLAN FOR JUNE 1st

|  | Planned | Unplanned |
|---|---|---|
| **Breakfast:** | ✓2 scrambled eggs | |
| | ✓2 slices turkey bacon | |
| | ✓1 large orange | |
| | ✓2 Tbsp nondairy liquid creamer in coffee | |
| **Snack:** | ✓6 oz flavored light yogurt | 12 almonds |
| **Lunch:** | ✓1 spinach salad | |
| | ✓5 ounces chicken breast | |
| | ✓1 slice whole-grain bread | |
| | ✓1 Tbsp brown mustard | |
| | ✓13 baby carrots | |
| | ✓10 small olives | |
| **Snack:** | ✓2 tsp peanut butter | |
| | ✓1 crispbread | |
| **Dinner:** | ✓1¼ cups vegetable soup | |
| | ✓1 cup spaghetti and meatballs | |
| | ✓13 asparagus spears | |
| **Snack:** | ✓1 cup halved strawberries | 1 extra cup of |
| | ✓⅔ cup frozen low-fat yogurt | frozen yogurt |

# Eating Guidelines

Use these guidelines as you transition into the Think Thin Initial Eating Plan:

## General Guidelines

**Prepare as many meals as possible at home; eat at home or carry your meals and snacks with you.** Restaurant eating requires special skills because many meals have double the portions you should eat or contain hundreds of hidden calories. You will greatly increase your probability of success if you focus on choosing and making Think Thin options at home—at least for the next few weeks, if not longer. Remember, you certainly don't have to eat at home for the rest of your life. But isn't it worth eating at home for a few weeks (which, in the course of a lifetime, is such a short amount of time) if it means you get to permanently keep off the weight you lose? Once you are firmly established on the Think Thin Initial Eating Plan, it will be much easier for you to handle restaurant eating and other challenging situations without experiencing a loss of control. During this time, if it's truly necessary to eat out, attend a social event, or travel, then by all means read ahead. You will find detailed advice for these types of challenges in Stage 3 (pages 127–166).

**Eat all of the food on your plan.** It's okay to leave food on your plate if you are full, but not if you are just trying to lose weight faster. If you routinely skip some food and find yourself getting hungry an hour later, this means you're not eating enough at meals.

**Notice your hunger level as you modify your eating.** If you are consistently hungry, do the following:

1. Make sure you are not confusing desire with hunger. Every time you want to eat something not on your plan, notice your sensations. Is your stomach empty? Then it's probably true hunger. Is the sensation somewhere else? Then it's probably not hunger.

2. Make sure you are not worsening the sensation of hunger by failing to respond to such sabotaging thoughts as, *This is awful ... I hate being hungry,* or, *Hunger is bad ... I should never feel hungry.*

3. Modify your eating schedule. Are you allowing too much time to pass between some of your meals and snacks? Try eating a snack or meal either earlier or later to see if that helps.

4. Make sure you're following the diet as laid out in the book. Are you skimping on protein or healthy fats?

5. For a few days at least, try changing to protein snacks.

**Create a weekly plan.** It is quite useful to take a few minutes, once a week, to think about the meals and snacks you will choose for the rest of the week. As best you can, try to plan the week's worth of breakfasts, lunches, dinners, and snacks. Make sure you have the ingredients you need or have a plan for when and how you will get them. When will you go to the grocery store? Are you often busy during the week? Would it be helpful for you to cook or prepare some food on the weekend for the coming week? A general weekly plan makes it so much easier; you'll have all of the food you need on hand. For example, if you planned grilled chicken for dinner one night and arrive home late after a busy day, it will be so much easier to stick to your plan if the chicken is ready and available.

## Food Selection Guidelines

**Use the options listed.** I've included simple, easy-to-prepare options to ease your transition into this new way of eating. If you still can't find enough food choices, read ahead to Stage 4 to learn how to modify your own recipes (pages 174–175).

**Eat less fat; get more food.** I've included the regular and reduced-fat versions for many foods. Selecting the lower-fat versions of foods give you a bigger portion and reduce your consumption of saturated fat, which has been shown to raise the risk of heart disease. Higher-fat versions of foods, however, may be more satisfying.

**Try as many options as you can.** Then narrow them down to a smaller group of meals that you really enjoy and can easily make. This simplifies planning and shopping.

**Designate a food preparation day.** Pick one evening or day (many spread it out over the weekend) to prepare and freeze a number of meal options. Also use this day to get a head start on planning some of the meal preparation needed for the week to come, such as chopping vegetables for salads.

**Create a supply of "safe foods."** Safe foods are convenient options that take very little preparation. Keep the ingredients you need on hand, continually updating your reserve, so when you've had a sudden change of plans, you can easily prepare one of these options. Whenever you cook, it's also

**tip:** Every time you measure food at home, look at the portion size. Notice how large it looks compared with your palm or fist. This will help you to better portion your food at restaurants and in other away-from-home eating situations. Also notice texture and color. This will help you to more easily spot the gleam of oil or butter on the vegetables served at restaurants or the overabundance of mayonnaise in tuna, seafood, or chicken salad.

a good idea to double or triple the recipe, freezing the remainder in individual portions to create your personal stash of "safe foods."

## Food Preparation Guidelines

**Use cooking spray.** This option saves lots of calories. If you'd like to cook with butter or oil, use your Add-On (page 225) or Bonus Calories (pages 226–227).

**Measure every portion.** For now, use a food scale and measuring cups and spoons whenever you are preparing a meal or snack. Don't estimate! Eventually you will get good at eyeballing your portions, but first you need to develop your eye.

When Greg began to measure his food, he realized that he had been serving himself considerably more food—especially meat and chips—than he had planned. No wonder he wasn't losing weight! I want to make sure this doesn't happen to you.

**Follow the plan precisely.** If the plan calls for you to use 1 teaspoon of olive oil and you use 1 tablespoon, you're adding 80 extra calories. If you eat 6 ounces of fried chicken when the plan called for 6 ounces of roasted chicken, you will add almost 200 calories. Half a cup of non-fat frozen yogurt is 110 calories, but having the same amount of ice cream adds 140 calories. Before you know it, your calorie count can vastly exceed the daily allotment. It's fine to use your Bonus Calories for an extra portion or extra ingredients, but make sure to plan for these calories in advance.

## Success Skills Guidelines

**Keep your Stage 1 skills sharp.** As some dieters transition into Stage 2 eating, they tend to lose sight of their Stage 1 skills. They may slide into eating some of their food standing up, or they may eat it too quickly or while distracted. They occasionally forget to read all of their Response Cards and Advantages Deck. Once they drift away from some of their Stage 1 skills, they always start making dietary mistakes. Your Stage 1 skills will help you to adopt and maintain your Stage 2 food plan. As you progress through this stage, *fill in your Stage 2 Success Skills Sheet (pages 268–269) every day.* It's an effective tool to ensure you keep yourself in check.

**Make time to prepare meals.** Will you need to

**tip:** To keep the ideas in your Advantages Deck fresh, go through the deck, select the three advantages that are the most important to you, and put these cards at the top of the deck. When you read the deck the next time, put those three on the bottom of the deck and pick the next three most important advantages. Doing this shuffle will make you focus more intently on the reasons you want to lose weight.

spend time in the evenings getting a start on your meals for the following day? Will you need to wake up early so that you can prepare breakfast or lunch? Don't forget that you may have to do some problem solving to create the time you need. But isn't it worth planning extra minutes into your day to ensure that you get to lose weight and keep it off?

**Don't forget to use your Food Plan Chart.** Write what you plan to eat for the whole day. Once you finish eating any meal or snack, immediately check off what you ate. Remember, don't be an ostrich with your head in the sand. Don't fool yourself! Every bite matters because with each decision about unplanned food, you're strengthening either your resistance muscle or your giving-in muscle.

**Use your Resistance Techniques** (pages 96–102). Immediately before eating, read your Response Cards so you will be prepared for any temptation. If you're tempted to eat something you hadn't planned to have, use your tactics. If you're still feeling tempted after a meal, try reading your Advantages Deck to remind yourself why it's so worth it to stop eating now. If needed, use Distraction Techniques. If you have trouble sticking to your plan, remind yourself that it will get easier and easier the more you practice your skills!

**If you make a mistake, don't catastrophize!** But do make sure to write the extra food in the "Unplanned Eating" column of your Food Plan Chart (page 91) and fill out a Cheat Sheet (page 104). Remind yourself that it doesn't make sense to continue to eat unplanned food for the rest of the day or even the rest of the meal or snack. Think about the red light analogy: Just because you ran one red light doesn't mean you should continue to run more.

**If you feel deprived after your meals, immediately read your Response Cards and Advantages Deck.** There are good reasons that you're not going to eat more! Also make sure you are still doing every Success Skill—especially eating slowly and enjoying every bite, as well as setting the timer for 20 minutes so you can see that fullness sets in. Remember, practicing these skills gives you more food satisfaction.

**Give yourself lots and lots of credit!** You deserve credit for taking the time to prepare meals; eating all of your food slowly, while sitting down and enjoying every bite; sticking to your plan precisely; and filling in your Food Plan Chart. Also *give yourself credit each time you resist eating something that wasn't on your plan.* Or if you do give in, give yourself credit for filling out your Cheat Sheet and getting back on track right away.

## Your Think Thin Breakfast Options

All of the Think Thin Breakfast Options (page 215) feature a significant amount of protein to help you feel full. In a study conducted at Saint Louis University, participants who consumed a dish rich in protein for breakfast reported feeling less hungry throughout the morning than participants who ate a dish rich in carbohydrates. That's why all of the breakfast choices on this plan—including the cereals—contain a significant amount of protein.

Do you prefer to eat sugar-sweetened cereal, breakfast pastries, refined bread, or baked goods for breakfast? The dieters I've counseled consistently report more hunger throughout the day after consuming such foods in the morning. These options just don't sustain them. Even though many of my dieters initially resisted having a high-protein breakfast, all of them were glad they switched once they discovered for themselves that their hunger was minimized and they had a much easier time following their eating plans.

If you need additional time to prepare or eat breakfast, do as much preparation as you can the night before. Or wake up earlier. Isn't it worth getting out of bed a few minutes sooner if it means you get to lose weight and keep it off?

**tip:** If you love a sugar-sweetened, low-protein breakfast cereal, you don't have to give it up. Eat it later in the day with your evening snack and count it toward your Bonus Calories.

## Your Think Thin Lunch Options

If you are progressing on the plan at the slow speed, I hope you have already begun to experience why this eating plan is so worth it—because it leaves you feeling satisfied, both in terms of the good food you eat and in the way it keeps you feeling fuller for longer.

All of the Think Thin Lunch Options (pages 216–217) feature lean protein to reduce hunger as well as hearty amounts of vegetables from salad, vegetable-based soup, or a vegetable side dish to help fill you up. Most vegetables are low in calories and high in water content. They weigh down your stomach, triggering stretch receptors to send the "I'm full" signal to the brain—which means you still feel full but you take in fewer calories. In a

**tip:** If you eat lunch at your desk, take some time to better organize your eating environment. Like a cluttered kitchen, a messy workspace loaded with books, papers, and reports can distract you and decrease your eating satisfaction.

Pennsylvania State University study, participants who consumed salad before lunch automatically ate less afterward than participants who did not eat salad. These researchers arrived at similar findings when participants started their meal with soup.

### Lunch Guidelines

Use this advice as you transition to the Think Thin Lunch Options:

**tip:** Many dieters find it useful to prepare some (or all) parts of their lunch ahead of time. For example, as soon as he returns home from the supermarket, Will immediately divides his big bag of baby carrots into individual portions to take with him as part of lunch each workday.

- All calorie levels of the plan include a side vegetable, salad, or soup with your meal. You will find basic salad recipes (page 219), reasonable vegetable portions (page 221), and a soup recipe (page 233). Don't choose higher-calorie soups or add extra toppings to your salad unless you plan them in advance. If a dish contains extra ingredients, you can use your Add-On Calories (page 225) or Bonus Calories (pages 226–227) for them.

- You can add one additional condiment or accompaniment (page 225) a day.

- Use cooking spray when pan-heating any lunch option.

- Consider using a spray margarine on your grain/starch or vegetables so you can use the calories you might have spent on butter for other foods.

- Consider using a spray salad dressing (10 to 15 calories per 10 sprays) on your salad or vegetables so you can use the extra calories for other foods.

## Your Think Thin Dinner Options

The Think Thin Dinner Options (page 218) include many simple, easy-to-prepare family favorites. You won't find gourmet, complicated recipes here for two reasons: First, at this point I want you to continue to spend your time and energy on making daily food plans, sticking to them, and continuing to practice your Stage 1 skills, not on preparing complicated dishes. Second, once most dieters start eating the foods on the Think Thin Initial Eating Plan, they discover that they actually like the taste of basic food. Until they started this eating plan, many of them had been accustomed to fried foods or foods with heavy sauces. Now, they find that they like the taste of simpler foods and like being able to eat larger quantities because they aren't spending the calories on additional ingredients. I think you may discover the same thing.

But if you are an accomplished cook or dedicated foodie, you can bring more complicated and lavish meals back into your life in Stage 4, which contains a set of gourmet recipes, along with advice for altering your personal recipes. For now, however, I encourage you to enjoy the simplicity of the Stage 2 dinner options.

Your Think Thin Dinner Options are all rich in protein and fiber to help fill you up on fewer calories.

## Dinner Guidelines

Use this advice as you transition to Think Thin Dinner Options:

- You can add one condiment or accompaniment (page 225) to dinner, if you haven't used one for a different meal.

- You will pair your main course with soup or a salad; a side vegetable; and a fruit or whole grain/starch, or both. See pages 210–214 for serving sizes that correspond to your calorie level. Use Add-On Calories (page 225) or Bonus Calories (pages 226–227) for extra ingredients.

- Use cooking spray for any dinner option that's cooked in a pan.

- Resist the urge to nibble as you cook. Don't fool yourself! Every calorie counts. It's okay to taste food for seasoning and flavor while cooking, if you need to, but don't consume more than that. Designate a teaspoon as a tasting spoon to keep on the counter while you're cooking. This will remind you that you're only going to use it once or twice—and only when necessary. Remember, if you spend calories tasting, you will have to reduce the calories you eat at dinner.

**tip:** Ask your family members to help prepare, serve, and clean up. Even children as young as four or five can learn to scrape their own plates.

- If you tend to eat extra food as you prepare dinner, consider having your afternoon snack just before preparing dinner to ward off hunger and temptation.

- Carefully measure your portion and plate it before sitting down to eat. Keep serving bowls away from the table. If they are out of sight, you will be less tempted to reach for seconds.

**tip:** If you're tempted to nibble as you store leftovers, ask family members to plate their food and then store the leftovers *before* you eat.

- Try using a smaller plate. It will make your portions seem larger so you will feel more visually satisfied.

- Designate time to make dinner. Again, preparation time doesn't automatically make itself available. Will you have time to prepare dinner just before eating? Many dieters like to get some of the prep work out of the way the evening or morning before.

- If you're tempted by food left on your family members' plates or in serving bowls, leave the kitchen! Don't return to the kitchen until your resolve is strong.

- Immediately after eating, scrape the plates and store leftovers. Make leftovers as difficult as possible to get to. For example, put refrigerated foods in opaque containers and place rubber bands around those containers; or wrap them in several layers of foil. Put them in the back of the refrigerator so they are difficult to see. Put other foods in a box with a lid or in a paper bag that you can staple shut. (Keep a stapler in the kitchen so you will remember to use it.) Having to open a box or undo staples gives you a chance to respond to sabotaging thoughts before you give in to eating. If you find you are continually tempted to eat leftovers, throw them away.

- After dinner, make sure your measuring cups and spoons are clean and ready to use the next day. Wash the dishes, clean the countertops, and get tempting foods under wraps and out of sight. Then leave the kitchen.

## Your Think Thin Add-On Options

You will select Add-On foods or ingredients from the list on page 225 for lunches and dinners. Choosing foods that contain fats will help you minimize hunger.

## Your Think Thin Snack Options

Your Think Thin Snack Options (page 224) are all healthy and high in protein and/or fiber to increase satisfaction and decrease hunger between meals. Eating snacks as planned is one of the hardest steps for many dieters because they often don't want to stop eating when they have finished their snack, or they want to be able to eat snacks other than the ones they planned. That's why it's so important to read relevant Response Cards and your Advantages Deck before eating your snacks, so that you can strengthen your resolve to follow your plan. Be prepared to use your Resistance Techniques, too, and remind yourself that you can always plan to have a favorite food tomorrow. Like all the skills and habits in this program, the more you practice, the easier it will be to stick to your snack plans.

## Snack Guidelines

Use this advice as you incorporate these snacks into your daily repertoire:

- It may take a little trial and error to find out which snacks work best for you. Try many different snacks from the list to see which leave you feeling the most satisfied.

- If you find you are consistently hungry between meals, choose higher-protein snacks.

- Change your mindset about snacks. If you want to lose weight and keep it off, you need to eat healthy snacks and limit "junk food" to no more than once a day.

- Each evening, measure out all your snacks for the following day and put them in "snack bags" to carry with you. Refrigerate the bags if they contain perishables. These snack bags will help you stick to your plan and avoid other foods, such as when you pass a vending machine, open a cabinet or refrigerator, or see a tasty treat in the breakroom. It's so much easier to resist these temptations if you know you have your planned snacks handy. When you get home from the supermarket, you might want to take snacks that come in a large quantity and prepare single-serving sizes to put in small containers or food storage bags.

## Your Think Thin Bonus Calorie Options

You have 150 or 200 Bonus Calories to spend every day in any way you wish. One wonderful aspect of Bonus Calories is that you never again have to feel guilty about eating a predetermined portion of your favorite foods. Many dieters are surprised when I tell them that they can use Bonus Calories for beverages or junk foods, such as alcohol; candy, chips, cake, or ice cream; sauces on their entrées; or butter. Previous diets had outlawed these beverages and foods.

It's important that you learn now how to eat your favorite foods in moderation. If you have the idea, *I can never eat cake again* (or whatever your favorite food is), you might be able to stop yourself from eating cake for a while. But sooner or later, you are likely to slip and have some. You might then have the thought, *I'll never allow myself to eat cake again, so I better load up now,* and end up eating a *lot* of cake. Knowing you can always plan to have your favorite foods the next day—and every day if you want—makes it easier to stick to your food plan. Results from Germany's Lean Habits study of 1,247 dieters bear out this idea. Dieters who tried to lose weight by eliminating sweets and other favorite foods were much less likely to maintain their weight loss than dieters who included these foods from the beginning of their diets.

Some dieters initially worry that they will lose control if they allow themselves to eat their favorite foods, especially sweets and salty snacks. I'm going to teach you how to gain control—even over your trigger foods!

I recently helped Mira introduce her favorite food back into her diet. She liked a certain sugary cereal, but she found that she had difficulty limiting herself to just one bowl. So she had decided to eliminate it from her diet completely. I asked Mira if she wanted to always ban this cereal or if she might like to have it some time in the future. She knew that she would want to eat it again at some point, so she decided to try to reintroduce it into her diet while she was still working with me. We devised a number of strategies: Right after Mira measured her bowl of cereal, she returned the milk carton to the refrigerator and put the cereal box back in the cupboard. When she finished eating, she immediately rinsed the bowl and spoon and put them into the dishwasher so she wouldn't be tempted to have more. She made some Response Cards, which she read before eating this snack, reminding herself why it was so worth it to eat only one bowl of cereal. Mira ended up making this card for her Memory Box:

> ### Memory Card
>
> I'm so happy! I can't believe I can finally eat my favorite cereal and stay in control. I can even have it every night if I plan for it. As long as I read my Response Cards, I'm fine. And the best part is that when I eat the cereal, it tastes so much better than it used to because I don't feel worried or guilty at all—so I enjoy every bite.

To gain control over trigger foods, plan to eat them with your evening snack, so you can look forward to the treat all day. Dieters find that it's easier to resist temptations during the day if they can say to themselves, *I don't want to eat this [unplanned] food now because I'd rather have my Bonus Calories tonight.* When it's time for your evening snack, measure out the portion you plan to eat and then immediately put the rest away. If possible, bring the snack out of the kitchen after dinner (assuming it's not something like ice cream) and declare the kitchen closed for the rest of the evening. Eat slowly, while sitting down and enjoying every bite.

Once you finish, brush your teeth and get involved in a distracting activity. If you want more after you have finished your treat, tell yourself you can have more tomorrow. Remind yourself that it's not terrible to wait, but you would feel terrible if you overate, lost control, and gained weight.

The first time you eat a tempting food with control and you find that experience particularly meaningful, file that in your Memory Box. This is the card Carol wrote:

---

### Memory Card

I didn't think I could hold myself to a single serving of ice cream. I was convinced I would lose control and eat the whole pint, but I didn't. I scooped a half cup into a small bowl, and I enjoyed every bite! I can do it!

---

## Bonus Calorie Guidelines

- If you are on the 2,200- or 2,400-calorie plan, you have 200 daily Bonus Calories. If you are on any of the other plans, you have 150 Bonus Calories.

- Don't make decisions on the spur of the moment about how to spend your Bonus Calories. Plan when and how to use them when you plan your meals and snacks.

- You can eat all of your Bonus Calories with one meal or snack, divide them up between two (or more) meals or snacks, or create an additional snack.

- Read Response Cards and your Advantages Deck before indulging in tempting Bonus Foods to remind yourself why it's worth it to stop after the planned amount.

- Over time, try to limit your consumption of foods with trans fat. It may be hard to give up these foods right now, but many researchers currently warn people against eating any trans fat because it has been associated with cancer and heart disease.

- In Chapter 10, on pages 226–227, I've included the portion sizes for many different possible Bonus Calorie foods. But you can use your Bonus Calories for any food or beverage; you are not limited to the suggestions on the Bonus Calories list. These are provided for your convenience, so you can easily find the correct portion size for a number of popular options.

- I've included Bonus Calorie suggestions for beverages, but most dieters find that they feel more satisfied if they use their calories on solid foods. Try low- or no-calorie beverages, such as water or tea. If you really like juice, experiment with diluting it 50-50 with water, gradually using more water and less juice over time so that you can save more of your Bonus Calories for solid foods. This is also a good strategy for switching from half-and-half to milk (or even skim milk) in your coffee.

## Graph Your Weight Loss

Now that you've started the Think Thin Initial Eating Plan, it's time to start graphing your weight loss. As I mentioned in Stage 1, many dieters expect their weight to continually drop, and they become frustrated when it periodically levels off or goes up. But it's important for you to know that *no one* loses weight day after day (or even week after week); it's a biological impossibility.

Even when you have been following your plan perfectly, it's likely that you will often step on the scale and see the same number appear for several days in a row. It's likely that your weight will often temporarily go up, even if you have been faithful to your eating plan. Maybe you ate more salt the day before so you are retaining water, or perhaps there is some other biological process going on. Weight loss may also halt when your body has reached a temporary set point. If you faithfully stick to your plan, your weight may drop again after a few days or weeks. If it doesn't, then it's time to step down to a lower-calorie plan or transition into maintenance.

Your weight may also stall once you start strength training. If you are working out vigorously, you can expect to acquire up to 3 pounds of muscle over a period of 12 weeks, which will show up on the scale as a gain. But you haven't gained fat, and the extra muscle will elevate your metabolism and can help you get past a weight-loss plateau.

I have found that most dieters understand these concepts intellectually, but they still panic whenever the number on the scale goes up. The only way to get over your panic is to graph your weight, day after day, and see that while there's a downward trend over time, on any given day the scale may have stayed the same or gone up.

If you haven't reached your final set point and if you are following the plan consistently, your weight will come back down, as Josie's did during the three weeks shown below as she progressed on the eating plan.

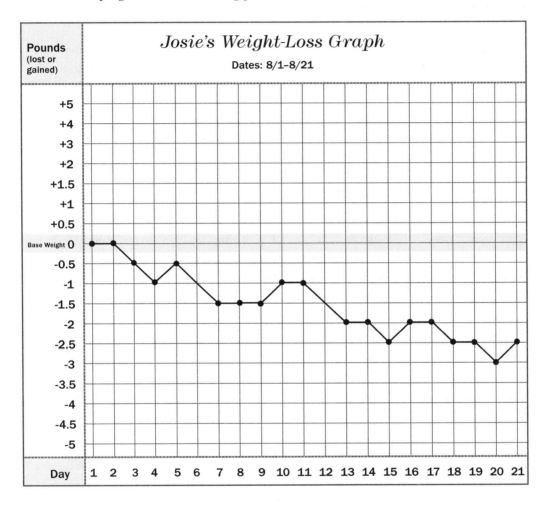

Without your graph, it's easy to let a small weight fluctuation ruin your day. When researchers at the University of Toronto weighed dieters on a scale rigged to show a false 5-pound weight gain, dieters reported a drop in self-esteem and mood and a rise in anxiety, guilt, sadness, and disappointment. They also ate more at a mock taste test than dieters who were told their true weight or a weight 5 pounds lighter than reality.

Are you ready to make your graph? Re-create the graph from page 265 on graph paper. (Or you can copy it in your Diet Notebook, photocopy it, or download it from www.beckdietforlife.com.) See the dot at the starting point? This indicates 0 pounds lost, which is where you were when you first started weighing yourself in Stage 1. Calculate the difference in your weight between then and today, and graph it. Did you gain a pound? If so, draw a dot on the Day 2 line that indicates +1.0 pounds. Did you lose half a pound? If so, draw your dot to indicate 0.5 pounds lost. Now, draw a line to connect the dots. Once you run out of room on this graph, create another one.

Every morning when you step on the scale and see the result, get in the habit of looking at your starting weight and telling yourself, *Since the beginning, the number on the scale is down by _____ pounds ... That is great!* Too often dieters get too focused on the number on the scale and fail to see the big picture. For instance, Mary had lost 10 pounds, but then, even though she was doing everything she was supposed to, the number on the scale went up by 2 pounds and stayed there for a week. She could have told herself, *Oh, I've been so good, but I gained 2 pounds anyway ... That's really terrible.* But she didn't. Instead, she said, *The number on the scale is down by 8 pounds since I started the program ... That's great ... I'm following my plan every day, and I'm exercising ... This is just a temporary blip, and I'm sure I'll start losing again ... But if I don't, I'll just change my eating.* Saying this to herself made it easy for Mary to maintain her motivation and to keep following the program.

## Before You Move On

Spend at least two to three weeks in Stage 2. Remain in Stage 2 until:

- You have successfully followed the entire Think Thin Initial Eating Plan (all meals and snacks) without any slips for at least two consecutive weeks.

- You have filled out the Stage 2 Success Skills Sheet and made contact with your Diet Buddy every night.

Remember, too, to continue to do as much spontaneous exercise as you can, to take a daily walk, and to do planned exercise—including strength training—on other days. To naturally lengthen the time you walk, consider wearing a pedometer—an inexpensive device you wear on your waistband that counts your steps. Women and men who wore pedometers for a Stanford University study naturally increased their daily walking by 2,183 steps—enough to cause them to lose an average of 3 pounds without changing their food intake. I have worked with several dieters who loved to record how many steps they took every day. They made it a personal challenge to figure out ways to add more. I also encourage you to start strength training twice a week if you aren't doing so already. You will find a simple, do-it-at-home strength-training routine on page 264.

As you get used to this new way of eating, it's normal to have a rebellious voice that urges you to return to your former choices and habits. You might miss larger portions. You might be tempted to eat whichever foods you want, whenever you want, without planning ahead. You might decide you don't have time to sit down to breakfast in the morning.

When you see yourself railing against the program, notice the thoughts that are running through your mind. If you have that voice that says, *I don't care … I'm going to eat it anyway,* remind yourself that this streak of rebelliousness is probably what has hampered you every time in the past. The rebellious voice is only concerned about what it wants right now. It refuses to consider how you're going to feel a few minutes from now and what the long-term consequences might be. You need to actually turn it on itself and rebel against your rebelliousness. Tell yourself, *I'm not going to let that voice get in the way … This goal is so important to me … I'm going to be so thrilled when I lose weight … I have to look at the bigger picture … Besides, listening to that voice has never gotten me where I want to be.*

And the longer you stay on the program, the more you will see your rebellious streak weakening as you:

- Give yourself credit for all of your positive eating behaviors.

- Feel proud of yourself.

- Realize how good it feels to be in control.

- Reduce your cravings for unhealthy foods.

- Feel satisfied with smaller portions.

- Experience the advantages from your deck.

- Feel virtuous, instead of deprived, when you resist unplanned food.

After a while, following your Think Thin Initial Eating Plan will become habitual. When you eat an unbalanced meal, you just won't feel as well. Time after time, I have heard dieters say that they lose their taste for their old eating choices. They say that following the Think Thin plan is now what feels good.

# chapter 6

# Stage 3

## The Challenging Situations Plan

During this stage, you will learn how to apply your Stages 1 and 2 skills when you eat outside the house, entertain at home, or are psychologically or physically stressed. For each challenging situation, you will develop a mindset that is different from your previous way of thinking and make specific Response Cards. Stage 3 will allow you to master these challenging situations:

- **Weekend Skills** (page 139)

- **Skills to Deal with Food Pushers** (page 141)

- **Restaurant Skills** (page 144)

- **Social Event Skills** (page 151)

- **Family Dinner Skills** (page 154)

- **Holiday Skills** (page 156)

- **Travel Skills** (page 160)

- **Skills for When You Are Under Stress** (page 163)

You will also learn additional skills that will enable you to successfully follow your eating program at restaurants, buffets, parties, special events, holiday meals, celebrations, hotels, and more.

During this stage, it's important to keep practicing all of your Stages 1 and 2 skills every day, even when you are not faced with a challenging situation; it's so easy to let these skills slip. For example, one day you may forget to prepare your snacks in advance (putting yourself at risk for snacking on unplanned foods). Another day, you might sleep late and not have time to eat breakfast slowly. Check off your Stage 3 Success Skills Sheet (page 270–271) every night to keep yourself on track.

## Summary of Challenging Situation Skills

Jot down this list of skills in your Diet Notebook under the heading "Challenging Situation Skills" so you can easily refer to it in the future. You will learn more about these skills on pages 131–164—and review this list many times in Stage 3:

Challenging Situation Skills

Before the Event:
1. Change your mindset.
2. Consult your Memory Box.
3. Develop an eating plan.
4. Review your Advantages Deck.
5. Create new and review old Response Cards.
6. Imagine the aftermath.

At the Event:
7. Use good eating habits.
8. Find an ally.
9. Use Resistance Techniques.
10. Give yourself credit.

After the Event:
11. Prepare for rebound desire.
12. Review the experience.
13. Use your Cheat Sheet (if applicable).
14. Weigh yourself tomorrow, no matter what.

It is important to read all of Stage 3 now, even if you don't expect any particular challenges to arise right away. I want you to be prepared.

## The Special Event Calories Decision

Right now you are going to make a very important decision about whether or not to have Special Event Calories. You can:

- Follow your Think Thin Eating Plan and keep your calorie count constant every day.

**OR**

- Eat up to 300 extra calories at a special event, as often as once a week (as long as you have planned to consume this extra food in advance).

There is no right or wrong answer. There are pros and cons to either option. If you keep your calorie count constant, it makes your life easier in many ways. You don't have to struggle with the decision of which day you are going to eat Special Event Calories. You don't have to remember when you last spent them. The rate at which you lose weight is a little faster, and you won't get in the habit of eating extra on some special days and possibly feeling deprived on other days. And, remember, you can always plan in advance to use your Bonus Calories at any event.

The second option offers you more choices when you go to a special event, *if you have planned in advance* to use your Special Event Calories. On these days, you will be able to add foods or beverages to your meal, in addition to Bonus Calories. But there are disadvantages to choosing this option: You will have to figure out the calorie content of the extra food or drink before you go to the event. You will still not be able to decide spontaneously to use your Special Event Calories. Also, some dieters can obsess for days: *Should I use my extra calories when we go out to dinner on Saturday night? Or should I use them at my cousin's party? And if I do use them, what should I spend them on?* For some dieters, having the choice makes their lives more difficult. They agonize over the decision, so for them it's better to forgo this option.

Another disadvantage is that it is sometimes difficult to stay within your Special Event Calories limit. A glass of wine can loosen your inhibitions, and you may start to eat extra food spontaneously. A piece of cake can spur a craving for more sugar. And some dieters start to feel resentful: *Why do I have to wait for a special event to eat more calories? Why do I have to limit the number of times I eat Special Event Calories each week or month?*

Another downside is that the extra calories can slow the rate of your weight loss a bit. Having Special Event Calories to spend works really well for some dieters—and not so well for others. You'll have to decide what is best and easiest for you.

Decide now what you want your rule to be. In your Diet Notebook, under the heading "Special Event Plan," record either:

- *It doesn't matter if there is a special event. I'm going to follow my regular Think Thin Eating Plan. I can plan in advance to use my Bonus Calories at the event if I want.*

**OR**

- *My rule for special events is:*

    * *I can have up to _____ extra calories.* (Fill in the blank with a specific number up to 300.)

    * *I can use my Special Event Calories up to once a _____.* (Fill in the blank with a time period between once a week and once a year.)

    * *I can use my calories at _____.* (Decide what constitutes a special event—a restaurant meal, party, conference, holiday, birthday, anniversary, etc.—and fill in the blank.)

If you choose the latter option, write down the following reminder, along with a system for remembering when you consume your Special Event Calories:

| |
|---|
| I can eat Special Event Calories only if I have planned in advance to have them for a specific event and I have also figured out the calorie content in advance. I can't use them spontaneously. |
| Every time I use my Special Event Calories, I will record the date [in my Diet Notebook or in my appointment book or PDA]. |

Whichever decision you make is not irrevocable. Try it out to see how well your rule works for you. If you run into difficulty, change it.

# challenging situation skills

You will now learn 14 skills that you will use over and over in Stage 3, particularly when you are eating out or entertaining guests at home. Practice them in each relevant situation:

## Before the Event

**1. Change your mindset.** In the past, did you ever think, *It's okay to make exceptions on weekends, holidays, or special occasions ... when I'm traveling, eating out ... when I'm stressed?* How well did this "It's okay to make exceptions" mindset work for you in your goal to lose weight permanently? The mindset of successful maintainers is different. They believe, *None of these exceptions matters ... Because I want to maintain my weight loss permanently, I'm going to eat in the same way 365 days a year (unless I have made a rule that it is okay to use Special Event Calories).*

If you're like many of the dieters I've counseled, you may be having the sabotaging thoughts, *But that's not fair! I want to be able to eat like everyone else ... I want to decide when to loosen up ... I just can't be as controlled in some situations as in others.* I always sympathize with the dieters, agreeing how unfair it is that some (actually only a few) people can eat whatever they want without consequences. But at least the unfairness of restricting one's eating pays off in all of the advantages of permanent weight loss.

In deciding to adopt this new mindset and to limit their food intake, dieters get so *much* in return. When they view the situation in this way, they come to realize that the trade-off isn't even close. They would much rather gain the benefits listed in their Advantages Decks.

So why *can't* you make exceptions? The fact of the matter is our body processes calories in exactly the same way whether we are home or out, whether it's a regular Monday or a holiday, whether we're working or on vacation. A calorie is a calorie, regardless of the situation in which you eat it. And if you make one exception, why not make more? Then you really put yourself at risk for gaining back weight. Just think: There are about 104 weekend days a year, not to mention the numerous holidays, anniversaries, birthdays, showers, weddings, parties, restaurant meals, fairs, conferences, meetings, special occasions, and vacation days.

Making exceptions also can lead to obsessing about your decision. *Should I make an exception for this party? Should I make an exception for that event?* Sticking to a predetermined rule takes the struggle and pain out of dieting.

I wish it were different. I wish *I* didn't have to be so careful every day. But I do (and so do all successful maintainers). And most of the time, I just don't think much about it because I know that the advantages of maintaining my weight are so much greater than the momentary pleasure of eating more on a special occasion.

Copy this Response Card and add it to your others:

> If I want to lose weight permanently, I can't make exceptions. I'd rather be thinner!

Many dieters initially feel they have to "get their money's worth" when they eat out. Or they have a hard time turning down free food. If you also have trouble with this way of thinking, make the following Response Card:

> "Free" food is only free in terms of money. Eating unplanned free food brings a heavy cost in terms of reinforcing my giving-in muscle and increasing my weight.

Do you have the unhelpful deprivation mindset I described on pages 45–46? A typical sabotaging thought is, *It's so unfair that I have to deprive myself.* If you think you might have that thought, make sure you continue to read the Response Cards that you made on pages 99–100. And create this new one, too:

I'm going to be deprived, no matter what. Either I'm going to be deprived of eating whatever I want at this special occasion OR I'm going to be deprived of being thinner, being healthier, feeling better about myself, being less self-conscious, being proud of myself, having more energy, and feeling good when the event is over!

**2. Consult your Memory Box.** Earlier in the day, read through the cards in your Memory Box. These memories can help motivate you for the upcoming event as you remember compliments and situations in which you were proud of yourself.

**3. Develop an eating plan.** After you read the cards in your Memory Box and fortify your resolve, decide what you are going to eat at the event. In Stage 4, you will learn how to be more flexible with your eating, adding your snack calories to a special meal if you like. But for now, I would like you to figure out what you are going to eat based on the Think Thin Initial Eating Plan and your Special Event Calories rule.

If you can, find out precisely what will be served and write down a specific plan. If you can't find out ahead of time which foods will be available, you will have to make a more general plan. On page 134, you will find a general plan, based on your Stage 2 dinner menu. Use this plan or create your own, making sure to keep to the same calorie level as your usual meal. Add it to your Diet Notebook under the heading, "General Plan for Eating Out." Note that I didn't include Add-On Calories. Most of the time, there will be extra fat in your meal that you don't know about.

**4. Review your Advantages Deck.** In addition to reading your deck each morning, pull it out immediately before going into a challenging situation. You may even need to take a break during an event and go outside or to a restroom to read it again.

It will be important to remember why it's worth it to stick to your plan when you encounter challenging situations. Try the following: Every morning, take the top

## General Plan for Eating Out

**Hors d'oeuvres or appetizer:** None, unless there are raw vegetables (without dip)

**Soup or Salad:** Make sure soup is a clear broth or consommé. (Most vegetable soups you are served will have too many calories.) If you prefer salad, make sure it resembles your basic daily salad and ask for dressing on the side. If there are extra ingredients (croutons, nuts, seeds, cheese, etc.), push them to the side so you won't eat them.

**Main course:** Plain protein, steamed vegetables, and one grain; ask for no sauce or sauce on the side and use minimally.

**Dessert:** None

**Bonus and Special Event Calories:** Decide in advance whether to use these calories, and, if so, how. (For example, you might have a glass of wine; a small piece of bread with butter; a small dessert; or an extra protein, grain, sauce, or dressing.)

three cards from your Advantages Deck or choose ones that represent benefits you have not yet fully achieved. Visualize the scene in detail: For example, imagine what a wonderful time you will have at your sister's wedding when you are slimmer and more self-confident, attractive, sociable, and at ease. Return those three cards to the bottom of the deck; next time, pull out the next three cards and do the same exercise.

**5. Create new and review old Response Cards.** Continue to read them each morning. If a challenging situation is coming up, take the most relevant cards and put them on top. If applicable, make new cards that apply to the particular situation. For example, Brian made the following card for his son's upcoming birthday party:

> I will feel so great when I stick to my plan at Max's birthday party. Eating extra will just make me feel weak and guilty. Besides, I want to be thinner at every single one of Max's birthdays in the future, so it's worth it to start now.

Immediately before — and during the event, if needed—read your Response Cards along with your Advantages Deck.

**6. Imagine the aftermath.** In Stage 1, you learned how to imagine the aftermath of a craving: the negative thoughts and feelings you would have after you gave in to a specific craving versus the positive thoughts and feelings you would have if you stood firm. Do the same with a challenging situation as a whole.

Immediately before you enter the challenging situation, imagine leaving it, having eaten too much. Can you see yourself feeling weak and defeated? Disappointed in yourself? Fearful of what the scale will show tomorrow? Unhappy about what you did? No longer confident in your abilities to lose excess weight and keep it off?

Then imagine that you are leaving the event, having exercised your resistance muscle and stuck to your plan. Can you see yourself feeling strong and in control? Looking forward to getting on the scale tomorrow? Happy about how you did? Proud that you proved you can stick to your plan during a challenging eating situation?

## At the Event

**7. Use good eating habits.** Don't make an exception about how you eat. It can be especially difficult to enjoy every bite when you are distracted by noise, conversation, and people walking around. Be sure to eat all of your food slowly, while sitting down and focusing intently on how it tastes. Otherwise, you can eat mindlessly and wonder, *Where did all my food go?* and be tempted to eat more.

**8. Find an ally.** Is there someone at the event in whom you can confide? Alert your ally in advance that you might need help if you have an intense craving. He/she could leave the room with you or distract you with conversation. Often just declaring aloud, "I'm not having any dessert," can be enough to exert the control you need to follow your plan.

**9. Use Resistance Techniques.** At the event, if you are tempted by unplanned food, do the following:

- Label what you're feeling at that moment: *I'm just craving/hungry/thirsty/tired/upset/ stressed/celebrating/happy.*

- Stand firm; tell yourself, *NO CHOICE ... I'm not going to eat this food.*

- Deal with disappointment: *Oh, well, I wish I could eat this but I can't, so I'm going to accept it and enjoy socializing ... I'm really going to enjoy getting and staying thinner.*

- Breathe deeply; relax.

- Distract yourself. Get involved in a conversation or activity.

- Go to the restroom or outside to read your Advantages Deck and Response Cards.

- Drink a no-calorie beverage.

- Distance yourself from the food.

**10. Give yourself credit.** Praise yourself at the moment for every positive eating behavior you use and for each instance of resisting unplanned food that tempts you.

## After the Event

**11. Prepare for rebound desire.** You also have to prepare to follow your plan after each challenging situation. Some dieters unravel when they get home and reward themselves for having been "so good." After Jan went to dinner with friends, she felt triumphant. While her friends consumed about 1,500 calories each, Jan stuck to her plan, stayed in control, and didn't become influenced by what the others were eating. On the way home, she told herself, *Look at all the calories I could have eaten and didn't!* When she got home, however, sabotaging thoughts kicked in: *I was so controlled tonight ... I deserve to have something else ... What can I have that would be healthy?* She ate a banana, some nuts, and two cheese sticks over the next hour and a half. It didn't seem like much, but these extra snacks put her over her daily calorie goal by several hundred calories—which slowed her weight loss and strengthened her giving-in muscle.

Jan was ready with this Response Card the next time she went out to dinner:

> It's worth it to me to stay in control at dinner. And I don't want to undo all of the good work I did at dinner by overeating when I get home. I'd rather be thinner!

**12. Review the experience.** Give yourself credit for everything you did right. If you made mistakes, write in your Diet Notebook (under the heading "Problem Solving for Future Special Events") what you can do to avoid future problems. If you had a positive experience, create a Memory Card describing the event, the skills you used, what you told yourself to stay in control, and how you felt afterward. These details will become your instruction manual for future real-life situations.

Stage 3 will bring lots of opportunities to create Memory Cards as you use your resistance muscle and feel good about staying in control. Maybe one will describe attending a social gathering and finding you enjoy yourself more than before because you aren't worrying about what you can and can't eat. Perhaps you'll create one when you feel triumphant instead of deprived because you didn't succumb to the high-calorie appetizers at a cocktail party. You might make a Memory Card when you leave a social event feeling elated and proud that you stuck to your plan—instead of feeling heavy, defeated, and sad because you didn't.

**13. Use your Cheat Sheet.** If you make a mistake, don't catastrophize. Don't criticize yourself or get discouraged. You're human. But learn from every mistake you make. The more often you use the Cheat Sheet, the more quickly you will be able to get back on track and the less likely you will be to make the same mistakes again.

**14. Weigh yourself tomorrow morning—*no matter what!*** If you eat food you hadn't planned, you may be mightily tempted to skip your weigh-in the next morning. It's critically important to get on the scale every morning without fail and not to stick your head in the sand. Remember, when has not getting on the scale every morning helped you lose weight and keep it off?

Elise had a history of yo-yo dieting. She was good at following her plan as long as she followed her predictable routine: eating most of her food at home, where she had control. But when she ate out and food was less controllable, she frequently made poor choices and overate; then she would continue to overeat when she came home. Afterward she would feel guilty and ashamed, sure that she had gained 4 or 5 pounds (a vast overestimation). She would avoid the scale for a week. Knowing she wouldn't weigh in for a while, she would loosen up. At the next weigh-in, the number on the scale often was up by several pounds.

Once Elise started weighing herself every day, she found two things: One, if she did make a mistake and overate one day, the number on the scale was only a pound or two more than the previous day, and she would lose this extra weight within a week. Two, it was far easier to get back on track immediately after arriving home than it was if she continued to overeat that night and in the following days.

The scale is one of the most important tools to help keep you accountable. Use it 365 days a year. But don't let a higher-than-expected number ruin your day. If you've made mistakes, don't criticize yourself. Just get problem-solving oriented. If you stick to your plan precisely, the number will undoubtedly go down soon.

## Confidently Follow Your Plan on Weekends

Weekends tend to be the downfall of many dieters. During the week, when they are focused on other tasks, they may not notice their hunger that much. But on the weekend, when dieters are less distracted, they may not only feel hungrier, but also have easier access to food if they're home and near the refrigerator. On the weekend, dieters also often have more unstructured time that allows them to think about eating, and they may have a greater desire to procrastinate doing a needed task and instead wander into the kitchen for food.

To consistently be successful on weekends, make the following special preparations:

### Create a Weekend Mindset

Do you view weekends as a break from work *and* a break from dieting? If your goal is permanent weight loss, weekends can't be considered a vacation from dieting. The most successful dieters and maintainers follow their diets consistently, no matter what day of the week it is. The National Weight Loss Registry, which follows thousands of maintainers, determined that study participants who consistently followed their diets—on weekdays *and* weekends—were 1.5 times more likely to maintain their weight loss over a year than dieters who loosened up on weekends.

Copy the following Response Card to practice a new mindset:

---

### WEEKEND RESPONSE CARD

Because I want to keep off excess weight, my weekend eating has to be the same as my weekday eating. My body doesn't know or care that it's a weekend, and if I eat too many calories, I'll gain weight. It's worth it to me to control my eating—even on weekends.

---

# weekend skills

Successfully following your eating plan during weekends takes more than a change in your mindset. In addition to practicing all of your other skills, you will need to use the following techniques (remember, the more you practice them, the easier they will get):

**Plan, plan, plan.** On Fridays or Saturday mornings, plan your meals for the entire weekend. Make your snack bags (described on page 120) and prepare any foods you might need in advance. Many dieters consistently prepare food ahead of time during the week because they know they need to pack meals or snacks to bring with them but forget that they need to do the same for weekends. Unfortunately, the food you need will not magically appear. If you spend time *every* day—and not just on weeknights—pulling together your snack bags and preparing other meals, you will be much less likely to relapse into spontaneous snacking on Saturdays and Sundays. Isn't it worth the extra preparation time if it means you get to lose weight and keep it off?

**Eat meals at structured times.** On the weekends, follow the same three-meals-and-three-snacks-a-day schedule that you use during the week. Many dieters are better off if they don't sleep late because it throws them off their eating schedule. If they have brunch (instead of breakfast and lunch), they often make up for the missed meal by having larger meals, larger snacks, or more snacks. Then when they go back to their usual schedule, they feel deprived. You can experiment with sleeping in, though, and see whether having brunch causes a problem for you.

**Get out of the house.** Structure your time, particularly in the beginning, to keep yourself from milling about in the kitchen. Plan to meet someone for a walk. Go on a family outing. Spend time doing yard work. Do errands.

**Create and use a non-food rewards list.** If you tend to splurge on Saturdays and Sundays because of sabotaging thoughts such as, *I worked so hard during the week ... I deserve to kick back and relax on the weekends,* then find non-food-related ways to reward yourself for your hard efforts. Consider taking a nap, relaxing in a hammock or hot bath, or getting a massage.

**Read your Response Cards and Advantages Deck more often.** You will probably need to read them several times a day to continually remind yourself why it's worth it to stay in control.

## Memory Box Cards

When you stick to your plan during a challenging weekend, create a new card for your Memory Box. Terry wrote:

> ### Memory Card
>
> I'm really glad I didn't overeat and didn't drink too much this weekend, like I did every time in the past when Ashley and Bob came to town. I felt really good this Monday morning. Thank goodness I made myself sit down on Friday to make a plan.

# Confidently Follow Your Plan Despite Food Pushers

Food pushers—people who offer food and strongly encourage you to eat it—can seriously sabotage your weight-loss efforts if you don't learn how to respond to them. Some food pushers try to make you feel guilty: "But I worked so hard to make this meal for you!" Some try to minimize the impact on your weight: "Oh, eating this one thing isn't going to make a difference." Some try to seduce you: "It's really, really good; you have to try it." Regardless of what the food pushers are saying, your response can always be the same: "No, thank you."

## Create a Food Pusher Mindset

To follow your plan when people suggest you do otherwise, you will need to respond to sabotaging thoughts, such as *I can't make her feel bad by turning her down,* or, *I can't stick up for myself.* Of course it's understandable that you don't want to disappoint another person, but you have to make a choice. Either *potentially* disappoint others and lose weight; or please them, strengthen your giving-in muscle, weaken your resistance muscle, and feel out of control, bad about yourself, and unhappy when you step on the scale. In short, disappoint *yourself.*

It's really okay—and important!—to turn down your aunt when she urges you to fill your plate with seconds or friends who enthusiastically encourage you to order another drink. It isn't rude to turn down people if you do so in a polite way. Ask yourself, *Why do I think I can't disappoint other people, but it's okay to disappoint myself?*

I have found that dieters tend to significantly overestimate how disappointed other people will be when they turn down offers of food—as well as how long other people's disappointment will last. Dieters are frequently amazed when a food pusher accepts their refusal and either changes the subject or tries to push the food on someone else.

Just think, if you ate differently from other people (and perhaps you do) because you were vegetarian, kept kosher, or had to follow a special diet for health reasons, you would *have* to turn down people when they offered you certain foods. It would probably be easier because you would feel entitled to do so. I'd like you to adopt the mindset that you are just as entitled as the people in those groups to decide what you are going to eat and what you are not going to eat.

If sticking up for yourself is a problem, make the following Response Card:

---

### FOOD PUSHER RESPONSE CARD

My goal to lose weight is more important than other people's momentary desire to have me eat their food. Their disappointment will likely be mild and brief. And it's so important to me to reach my goal.

---

# skills to deal with food pushers

Once you feel comfortable with the idea of saying no, you're ready to create a plan. First, make a rule that you will not eat when someone offers you food that you haven't planned for—*no matter what*—unless you really want to take the food home and plan to have it another day. But if you think you'll be tempted to eat it before you plan to, don't take it with you; you'll regret eating it. Second, if food pushers push food on you, just say, "No, thank you," and then quickly change the subject. If they persist, you can also persist by sounding like a broken record: Just keep saying, "No, thank you. No, thank you. No, thank you." If they ask why you're turning down the food, you don't have to give a reason. You can simply say, "I just don't want it now. But thanks, anyway."

# in session with Dr. Beck

Anna was able to stick to her eating plan in almost every situation except when people offered her food. Anna believed she was entitled to follow her plan, but she had a difficult time being assertive.

**Dr. Beck:** Who is the hardest person to turn down?

**Anna:** My mother-in-law.

**Dr. Beck:** Could we role-play? You play your mother-in-law, and I'll be you. Offer me something to eat.

**Anna** *[as her mother-in-law]:* Anna, come have a piece of the pie I made.

**Dr. Beck** *[as Anna]:* Oh, thanks, but no, thank you.

**Anna** *[as her mother-in-law]:* Don't tell me you're dieting again! You know you won't lose weight.

**Dr. Beck** *[as Anna]:* Oh, well, I'm afraid I have to say no, thank you. [changing the subject] Have you made any holiday plans yet?

**Anna** *[as her mother-in-law]:* [ignoring the question] Come on, you can have a taste. I spent all day cooking it for you and Rick.

**Dr. Beck** *[as Anna]:* Oh, that was nice, but no, thank you.

**Anna** *[as her mother-in-law]:* If you don't try it, you'll hurt my feelings.

**Dr. Beck** *[as Anna]:* That's not my intention, but I have to say no, thank you.

**Anna** *[as her mother-in-law]:* Come on, you can at least have a taste of it!

**Dr. Beck** *[as Anna]:* No, thank you.

**Anna** *[as her mother-in-law]:* But it'll go to waste!

**Dr. Beck** *[as Anna]:* No, thank you.

**Anna** *[as her mother-in-law]:* I can't understand why you can't at least try it.

**Dr. Beck** *[as Anna]:* No, thank you.

**Anna:** [pauses] I don't know what she would say next. I think she'd probably finally leave me alone.

Next, we discussed Anna's concern that her mother-in-law would get mad and stay mad at her. Anna told me that her mother-in-law is constantly finding fault with Anna and seems continually annoyed at her. Anna concluded that her mother-in-law probably wouldn't be much more annoyed than usual as a result of the pie incident.

### Memory Box Cards

If you are proud of yourself for being assertive with a food pusher, write a card for your Memory Box. Kirk wrote:

> **Memory Card**
>
> I can't believe I was finally firm with Mom. She seemed a little shocked when I insisted I wasn't going to have her twice-baked potatoes. But she didn't make a big thing of it. I'm glad I stuck to my guns! And now I know I can do it again the next time.

## Confidently Follow Your Plan at Restaurants

Following your plan at a restaurant takes preparation and practice. Learn how to manage in this environment, and it will be easier to eat in other challenging situations as well.

### Create a Restaurant Mindset

Typical restaurant servings in America are double or triple what most people can eat and maintain a healthy weight. No wonder researchers at Queens College of the City University of New York found that people tended to consume more calories when they ate out and that people who ate out often tended to weigh more than people who mainly ate at home. University of Pennsylvania researchers have determined that people who live in areas densely populated by restaurants—particularly fast-food restaurants—tend to weigh more than people who live in areas with fewer options.

It's important that you start viewing restaurant meals for what they really are: abnormally large. If you don't, you will feel deprived when you can eat only part of what you are served. When you get your meal and portion off the part that you can eat, tell yourself, *This is a normal portion for a successful dieter or maintainer.* Remind yourself that it's worth it to forgo that extra food if it means you get to lose excess weight and keep it off. Besides, you can always wrap up the extra food and plan to have it the next day—that way you get to enjoy two meals from it.

I want you to feel entitled to make special requests. If you had a serious health problem, you wouldn't think twice about asking for food to be prepared to your specifications. I had to do this for several years whenever we ate out with my son, who was on a special ketogenic diet for epilepsy. His diet required he consume a strict ratio of four parts fat to one part protein and carbohydrates. We had to ask for his food to be prepared in a special way. We had to bring his beverage and a food scale to restaurants and then weigh every gram he ate. I never felt embarrassed—not at a fast-food restaurant, not at a fancy restaurant—because it was simply what we had to do for his health.

Are you thinking, *Yes, but you had a legitimate reason to make special requests?* If so, I want to remind you that your goal to lose weight and be healthy is legitimate, too. You're also entitled to send food back if it's not prepared in the way you ordered.

You should not hesitate to speak up. If you have the sabotaging thought, *I don't want to make trouble,* or, *I'm being high maintenance,* tell yourself that people make special requests at restaurants all the time. The wait staff won't be surprised. Just be sure to tip them a little extra if they go out of their way for you.

Create the following Response Card to help you follow your plan at restaurants:

---

### RESTAURANT RESPONSE CARD

If I want to successfully eat at restaurants, I have to follow my usual eating plan, make special requests, waste food, and remind myself that successful dieters and maintainers do exactly the same thing.

---

# restaurant skills

You won't always have to put as much effort into practicing the skill of eating out because it gets easier. Until it does, however, you will have to make an extra effort. For your first eating-out experience, it's a good idea to dine with a companion who either knows you are dieting or who doesn't push food on you. If possible, eat with your Diet Buddy. Also, choose a restaurant with a menu you can check out ahead of time. If the menu isn't available online, have it faxed to you or stop by beforehand to pick one up.

Choose items that correspond to the Think Thin Initial Eating Plan. Use your Think Thin Food Lists (pages 215–227) for guidance. Design your meal and figure out portion sizes you can have without going over the calorie limit for this meal.

At the beginning of this chapter, I described a basic restaurant menu that included a green salad or consommé, lean protein, steamed vegetables, a side of grain, and suggestions for using your Bonus Calories (page 134). Below are some additional main-course menu ideas (start each meal with a salad with no extras and dressing on the side):

- One and a half slices of plain, thin-crust pizza and a side of steamed vegetables. Count the crust as your grain serving and your Bonus Calories, if needed. Blot excess oil off the pizza with a napkin before eating.

- A veggie or turkey burger or a small-sized hamburger with half of an unbuttered bun or a very small portion of French fries and a side of steamed vegetables. Ask for condiments on the side because burgers sometimes come with mayonnaise or a mayo-based sauce.

- Pasta primavera (sauce on the side) with a source of protein (shellfish, chicken, or fish) mixed in and a side of vegetables. Count the pasta as your grain serving and your Bonus Calories, if needed.

- Chinese chicken or shrimp with vegetables. Ask for the chicken or shrimp and vegetables to be steamed and served without any oil. Ask for rice and sauce on the side. Get brown rice if it's available and mix only ½ cup into your meal (counting it as your grain serving). Use minimal sauce, counting it as your Add-On Calories or Bonus Calories, as needed.

- Tandoori chicken with a vegetable side dish, such as eggplant or peas, or a bean side dish, such as lentils. Indian food is often cooked with calorie-laden sauces. If you can't get sauce on the side, count those extra calories as both your Add-On Calories and Bonus Calories.

- Japanese sushi or sashimi (use portions suggested in the Think Thin Food Lists on pages 216–218) with miso soup and seaweed salad. Count the rice as a grain serving.

Beware of options that *sound* reasonable but may not be as healthy as they seem. For example:

- **Burritos:** Because burritos are flour or corn tortillas mostly stuffed with protein, vegetables, and rice, many dieters fail to estimate their true calorie count. Certain ingredients—especially rice, cheese, guacamole, avocado, sour cream, and sauce—

add lots of calories. Many restaurant burritos are also enormous, with some totaling more than 1,000 calories. Just the tortilla alone may contain 300 calories.

- **Chef, Cobb, or taco salad:** Ingredients such as eggs, avocado, olives, nuts, seeds, dried fruit, croutons, bacon, cheese, Chinese noodles, tortilla strips, and dressing can drive up the calories, with some jumbo salads totaling more than 1,000 calories. The large serving of shredded cheese that tops some restaurant salads comes to more than 400 calories by itself. The fried tortilla bowls that taco salads are often served in may have several hundred calories.

- **Chicken or tuna salad:** The amount of mayonnaise used in these dishes makes a huge difference and can total 200 or more calories.

- **Sandwiches:** Creamy dressings and spreads can run up the calorie count by more than 200 calories. The type of bread used makes a difference, too—with thicker focaccia bread or hoagie rolls adding hundreds of extra calories.

- **Fruit smoothie:** You can make wonderful fruit smoothies at home. Smoothies served at many restaurants are usually larger than homemade ones and may contain more than just fruit, water, and yogurt; they are often loaded with sugar and/or high-fructose corn syrup. Some commercial smoothies actually contain more sugar than some types of doughnuts—and total more than 500 calories.

If you hadn't done your research ahead of time, you might have mistakenly thought that these options were low in calories. Watch out for foods that are described as fried, pan-seared, or sautéed, because they will be prepared in oil. Also be on the alert for food that is breaded—for example, shrimp, pork chops, veal, or chicken. If in doubt, ask. You don't want to be surprised by a high-calorie dish—because you will have to eat much less of it.

## Before You Go

Use all of your Challenging Situation Skills. Before you leave for the restaurant, plan what you are going to eat, consult your Memory Box, review your Response Cards and Advantages Deck, and imagine the aftermath.

## At the Restaurant

**Make special requests.** Your meal will undoubtedly contain extra calories in the form of sauces, cooking oil or butter, and even sugar. For example, eggs are cooked in butter unless you ask for them to be prepared with cooking spray. Many restaurants put butter or mayonnaise on their burger buns. Most entrées come with 1 to 2 tablespoons of added oil. That's an extra 100 to 200 calories! You can use your Add-On Calories or Bonus Calories to account for these ingredients, or you can request that your food be served free of sauces and oils—or, at the very least, with the sauces on the side. Or be prepared to eat smaller portions.

I encourage you to ask for:

- **A low-calorie salad dressing alternative,** such as balsamic or red wine vinegar, salsa, or a wedge of lemon, unless you want to ask for salad dressing on the side and use your Add-On Calories or Bonus Calories for it. Or bring a packet of your favorite low-calorie dressing or salad dressing spray with you. Remember, if you had to follow a special diet for medical, religious, or philosophical reasons, you wouldn't hesitate.

- **Your vegetables to be steamed and served without any oil or butter.** Ask for extra veggies if none or few come with your entrée. Be willing to pay extra for these. Most restaurants are willing to serve you salad in place of French fries, for instance, or broccoli in place of rice or pasta.

- **Your protein (fish, seafood, poultry, lean beef, pork) grilled or broiled,** with no sauce, butter, or oil. If you want to use your Bonus Calories for sauce, ask for it on the side *if you have figured out ahead of time how much of it you can have.*

- **Your grain plain,** unless you want to use your Add-On Calories or Bonus Calories for butter, sauce, or a different topping. Be forewarned: Restaurants routinely add butter or cream to such foods as mashed potatoes and rice to make them taste better. You won't know, though, unless you ask.

- **Fresh fruit for dessert, if your plan allows for it.** Many restaurants have fresh berries or other fruits, even if they don't mention it on the menu. Just make sure to ask that the fruit be served plain—without whipped cream, sauce, or powdered sugar.

**Assess your food.** Are vegetables glistening, even though you requested no butter or oil? Do veggies or starches taste richer than they do at home? If so, assume your special request was not granted; don't hesitate to send food back to the kitchen.

**Portion off the extra.** Before you take your first bite, separate the portion you are supposed to eat from the rest of the food on your plate. Estimate the size of your portion on the low side; there are likely to be some hidden calories in your food.

**Eat slowly and enjoy every bite.** This practice is especially important if you are dining with companions. If you are the last person to finish eating, you will be much less tempted to eat more. Make sure to really savor your food.

When you dine out, you are practicing multiple skills at once: You're learning how to stand firm in the face of temptation, how to be assertive, and how to waste food. It's normal to make mistakes at first. Fill out a Cheat Sheet and use each mistake as a chance to improve your subsequent experiences. Remind yourself that the more you practice these skills, the easier restaurant eating will get.

### Memory Box Cards

When you have meaningful restaurant experiences, write cards for your Memory Box. For example, this is a card Kim wrote:

---

Memory Card

I've been trying to get over my embarrassment of bringing my own salad dressing with me to a restaurant. Yesterday when I went out to eat with Vanessa, I finally brought the dressing. I thought she would be critical of me, but instead she thought it was a great idea.

---

## Special Advice for Buffet Restaurants

As you go along, choose progressively more challenging types of restaurants or cuisines and, if at all possible, save the most challenging of all—buffets and cafeteria-style restaurants—for your last challenge. Buffets are particularly problematic because of the wide variety of foods offered. It's tempting to put small amounts of lots of different foods on your plate, but these small amounts usually add up to many more calories than your plan budgets for. And dieters often find that many small tastes leave them feeling less satisfied than larger portions of fewer foods.

When you practice the art of buffet eating, do the following:

- Stick to your usual plan (as you would for any restaurant).

- Decide whether you will use Bonus Calories for this meal.

- Remind yourself that trying to "get your money's worth" will cost you a lot in terms of gaining weight and strengthening your giving-in muscle. Isn't the goal of getting thinner, with all its accompanying advantages, much more important?

- Walk around the buffet before putting anything on your plate, reminding yourself of your pre-planned options.

- As you plate your food, give yourself credit for choosing foods that are on your plan.

- If your choices are glistening with butter or oil or are covered in a sauce, take a smaller portion than you would if you'd prepared the dish at home and scrape off as much of the sauce as you can.

- Wait until you sit down to eat your first bite of food. It's easy to eat hundreds of calories while you're still in the buffet line; food eaten this way won't satisfy you enough, will reinforce an unhelpful habit, and will leave you with less food to eat once you sit down.

- Don't go back for seconds. If you feel tempted, read your Response Cards and use Resistance Techniques.

## Special Advice for Ordering In

Follow the same guidelines for take-out foods as you would for eating out. Don't be afraid to speak up if your entire family or the friends you have over want to order food that doesn't correspond to your plan. Feel entitled to order what *is* on your plan.

If the leftovers are tempting, put them inside a brown paper bag, staple the bag, and store it in the back of the refrigerator. If they are still too tempting, even with the extra packaging, throw them out. Remember, the food will go to waste either in your body or in the trash can. I often hear from dieters that they are the only ones who really eat the leftovers anyway. So I suggest that they just go ahead and throw out the leftovers right away if they don't want to end up eating them or if they can't think of when they will plan to eat them.

**The more often you practice eating out and ordering in, the better you will get at it.** You will make a shift from, *I feel deprived,* to, *I'm so happy I stuck to my plan.* You will also make a shift from, *I can't wait to eat a lot,* to, *I'd so much rather be thinner* *than eat extravagantly ... It's not worth it!* Eventually, making special requests will no longer feel difficult. You will naturally ask for what you need and will no longer confront as many sabotaging thoughts. You will also start to automatically make smarter choices and learn to recognize hidden calories.

Having said all that, if you eat out a lot and find that you are not losing weight (or you are gaining), it's likely that:

- The portions you consume are too large.

- There are hidden ingredients that you are not counting.

- Your special requests are not being honored.

- The restaurant has supplied you with misleading information. A Center for Science in the Public Interest analysis determined that some restaurants served meals that contained hundreds more calories than what was listed on their menus.

- You may have to eat out less often. Remember that eating in saves you calories— and money.

# reality check

**If you are thinking:** *It's okay to go off my diet because I'm at a restaurant. Besides, everyone else is eating this way.*

**Face reality:** It doesn't matter how much everyone else eats. Whatever calories someone else puts into his/her body has absolutely no effect on the calories you put in *your* body. Remember, it's your goal to lose weight and keep it off, so you're responsible for making it happen.

## Confidently Follow Your Plan at Social Events

Many dieters tell me they sometimes avoided or dreaded social gatherings. They thought there was no way to say no to birthday cake without feeling deprived or guilty. They didn't think they could go to a bar and forgo the free snacks or extra drinks. They especially feared parties where hors d'oeuvres were offered, not to mention a heavy main course with dessert.

I never want you to avoid a social event for fear that you will overeat! These events are an extension of eating out, and you will use many of the skills you used for restaurant eating. The more you practice, the easier these situations will become.

I know dieters who initially thought it was impossible to stay in control at social events; but the more they practiced and learned from their mistakes, the better and better every one of them became at this kind of challenging situation.

### Create a Social Eating Mindset

Put the "social" back in social events. Think of them as *people* events—as a chance to catch up or meet someone new. If you feel deprived, remind yourself that if you overeat, you will be deprived of feeling in control, good about yourself, proud when you leave the event, and happy when you get on the scale the next morning. If you fool yourself into thinking it is okay to change your eating plan at the last minute, ask yourself how well making spontaneous food decisions has worked in the past. Overeating at social events strengthens your giving-in muscle and is likely to make it harder to stay on track, exert self-control at the next event, and, ultimately, lose weight. Keep reminding yourself that you're not being deprived of *all* food, and you get so many advantages in return.

Read this Response Card before attending a social event:

> ### SOCIAL EVENTS RESPONSE CARD
>
> I need to make social events be about the people and not about the food. I have to face the fact that every time I eat spontaneously at a social event, I undermine my efforts by strengthening my giving-in muscle. Every time I stick to my plan, I feel great and in control.

# social event skills

To handle social events with ease, you will use many of the skills already presented in this chapter. Here are some additional suggestions:

**Bring food with you when you can.** Depending on the type of event, you may be able to bring foods you can eat. Jacob planned to take turkey burger patties and a salad with him to a barbeque. Another time, he brought two desserts to a dinner party: fruit that was on his plan and a cake he didn't particularly like.

**Eat smaller portions, if necessary.** What do you do if there are no options that are on your plan? Eat less than you ordinarily would eat at home. You've already proven to yourself that hunger is not an emergency.

**Sit down to eat.** You just won't be able to appreciate every bite if you eat while standing. If there aren't any chairs, be creative. What would you do if you had a broken leg? You'd have to find a place to sit down. Perhaps you can find a step to sit on or ask for a chair.

*************

I don't expect you to be perfect the first time you go to a social event. As with eating out, social events require you to practice many skills at once. You may make mistakes at first. But practice makes perfect, and you *will* improve. You will transition from thinking, *It's so unfair that I couldn't eat what I wanted,* to the liberating thought, *I'm so glad I don't have to worry about losing control of my eating at social events ... I can just go and have a good time.*

## Memory Box Cards

The first time you stay in control at one of these events and find it meaningful, file that experience in your Memory Box. For example, Laurie wrote:

> ### Memory Card
>
> I went to Kevin's football party. He served pizza, wings, and lots of chips, but I stuck to my plan. I used my skills, stayed in control, and felt great! Now I know I can eat pizza and stay in control. It's such a great feeling!

**How wonderful it is to go to bed after a special event or celebration and feel so good that you followed your plan,** when you could have easily consumed thousands of extra calories.

## Special Advice for Entertaining at Home

Some dieters find it easier to stick to their plan when they host a special event at home where they control what is served; some find it harder because they have to spend more time thinking about, shopping for, preparing, serving, and clearing away the food.

Here are some ideas for you to consider:

**Have a firm plan.** Avoid making spontaneous decisions. Read your Response Cards and Advantages Deck ahead of time to remind yourself of the reasons it's worth it to stick to your plan.

**Change the food you serve.** Offer healthy choices that you can eat. So many people are health conscious these days; your guests are likely to be grateful that you are serving delicious, wholesome food that makes them feel good instead of overstuffed and guilty. And if you find a particular food or dessert too tempting, don't serve it!

**Request help.** Ask a friend or family member who is coming to your house to arrive early to help you prepare and set out food. Ask someone else to stay late to help you put away extra food and clean up. Be extra careful to resist rebound desire after the party. It's not worth it to overeat once everyone has left.

**Take time to eat properly.** Sometimes hosts get so busy that they pick at food all night instead of having a proper meal. Make sure to sit down, eat slowly, and enjoy every bite.

**Give away the leftovers.** Have containers and food storage bags on hand, and ask people to take the extra food that you think will be too tempting.

## Confidently Follow Your Plan at Extended Family Dinners

Family dinners require you to combine skills from social events and holiday eating (pages 155–157). You will also have to learn how to stay true to your plan in the face of strong emotions—either positive or negative. You will need to be really good at saying no to food pushers (pages 141–143), too, as some families have strong beliefs about food and eating. For example, your family members may comment on the foods you are eating or not eating, complain that you are eating differently from them, or try to ply you with alcohol.

### Create a Family Dinner Mindset

When adults spend time with their families, they sometimes revert to old patterns of thinking and behaving—and sometimes start feeling like children again. To help maintain your mature, adult mindset, read a Response Card such as the following:

---

#### FAMILY DINNER RESPONSE CARD

I need to decide what is right for me to do and what is right for me to eat, even if it bothers other people. I may feel more emotional (either positively or negatively) than usual, but it's so important for me to stick to my plan anyway and to prove to myself that I can absolutely stay strong.

---

# family dinner skills

Try the following strategies:

**Fortify your resolve before you go.** Expect that this meal may be more difficult than normal and that you may have to work harder to stay in control.

**Feel entitled.** Bring one or more dishes that you know you can eat. You don't necessarily have to announce in advance that you're doing this.

**Be assertive.** Do what you need to do. Nicely say, "No, thank you," if someone pushes food or drink on you. Change the subject if someone starts talking about your eating, weight, or appearance, and you would rather not discuss it.

**Take a walk.** Excuse yourself and walk around the block if you find you're getting too stressed or tempted.

**Do deep breathing.** If things get tense, take relaxing breaths (instead of a drink).

**Defuse the tension.** A little humor goes a long way when things are tense. Make light of others' critical comments. Let them roll off your back.

### Memory Box Cards

The first time you follow your plan during a family dinner and find that experience particularly meaningful, file it in your Memory Box, as Heather did:

---

**Memory Card**

Today was Dad's birthday. Mom criticized me a lot for not eating the birthday cake she had made. But I didn't care! I didn't even feel like I had to take a piece of cake home just to appease her. I remembered that I'm in control of what I eat! I'm just not going to eat what she wants me to—ever—unless I decide to do so.

---

## Confidently Follow Your Plan During Holidays

Holidays are difficult. Some of the difficulty is practical: We run around, we have less time, we're exposed to food at every turn. Some of the difficulty is psychological and requires a mindset change.

### Create a Holiday Mindset

While many people are busy preparing for and celebrating holidays, they begin to have sabotaging thoughts, such as:

- *It's okay to stop scheduling time for my dieting and exercise activities.*

- *I should be able to live it up a little.*

- *I'm too busy.*

- *I don't have to plan what I'm going to eat because I'm just going to try to maintain my weight. I'll just be careful.*

- *I'm going to skip my daily weigh-ins until after the holiday.*

Left unchecked, these thoughts can cause serious damage. To follow your plan during holidays, accept the reality that you can't eat the way you used to *if* you want to get and stay thinner. It doesn't matter that it's holiday time; others are eating and drinking a lot; you're exposed to special food; or your host is pushing you to eat more. *If you eat extra calories, you are going to gain weight.* Remind yourself that you have a choice: You can give in to holiday temptations, or you can practice these skills and keep the excess weight off for good. If you choose the latter, it's true you will be giving up eating some food. But you will be getting so much in return. Ask yourself: *Where do I want to be next holiday season? And the season after that? And the season after that?* If you always want to be a thinner, healthier, in-control person, it's essential for you to learn these skills now. Then you will be able to use them at every future holiday. Create this Response Card to read each morning around a holiday:

---

### HOLIDAY RESPONSE CARD

My body doesn't know it's the holidays. Holiday time is not a reason to eat unplanned food. When the holiday is over, I'm going to be so glad that I stuck to my plan. It's worth it to forgo the momentary pleasure of eating foods I haven't planned to eat so I can stay in control, be happier with myself, and lose weight.

---

# holiday skills

Just as social events are an extension of eating out, holidays are an extension of social events. Here's what to do:

**Create a general holiday plan.** You may attend many events during some holidays. Rather than create a specific plan for each event, you can have one general plan for all of them. You might decide, for example, to use your Bonus Calories toward a glass of wine or small dessert whenever you go out to a holiday function. Beware of the dangers of having no plan (*I'll just try to limit myself*), too loose of a plan (*I'll just have a little bit of some things*), or having a plan but not following it (*It won't hurt if I have this food I hadn't planned to eat … I can always start again tomorrow*). These sabotaging thoughts are likely to result in gaining weight.

**Create holiday rules.** Think about situations that have tempted you to overeat and feel guilty in the past. Then create reasonable rules, such as, "I will not eat any goodies that people bring into my office," or, "I'll use my Bonus Calories for office goodies if I want to, but I'll bring the right portion home and eat it with my evening snack." Having such rules makes avoiding unplanned food so much easier and less painful because, when confronted with such food, you never have to go through the struggle that makes dieting so difficult: *Should I eat this? I know I shouldn't ... But it looks really good ... But it's not on my plan ... But it's so hard to resist....* When you automatically say to yourself, *I'm definitely not going to have any ... NO CHOICE,* you eliminate the struggle and move on.

**Talk yourself through temptation.** Remind yourself that if you hadn't seen holiday goodies, you may not even have thought of them or wanted them. This helps diminish your sense of entitlement. If you say to yourself, *I only want [this food] because I'm seeing it right now, but I can move on as if I'd never seen it,* it will be easier to resist.

### Memory Box Cards

Holidays are perfect occasions for storing important memories so you can motivate yourself in the future. Here's what Scott wrote on his card:

> ### Memory Card
>
> It was hard to resist the cake and ice cream at the [holiday] party today, especially since most people were eating them. But now that it's over, I'm glad I did. It would have been much harder if I hadn't read my Response Cards before I went and made a rule about not having any beer. I remember how guilty I felt last year after this same party.

## Confidently Follow Your Plan While Traveling

Traveling can be a challenge: You have less access to the foods you usually eat. Getting to your destination can be stressful. Your usual routine is disrupted, mealtimes may be irregular, and you will likely be exposed to tempting foods and drinks. Some dieters find it relatively easy to keep up their efforts for a few days but then slip into loose eating and gain weight. To avoid this pitfall, change your mindset about traveling.

**Create a Travel Mindset**

You just can't take a vacation from dieting without regaining weight. Not responding to the following sabotaging thoughts will make traveling difficult and gaining weight probable: *I can't stick to my diet ... I shouldn't have to stick to my diet ... I don't want to stick to my diet.* While you may not have control over foods, you should plan to follow the Think Thin Eating Plan as best you can, eating the usual number of calories for each snack and meal. If you wish, you can supplement this plan with extra Travel Calories (at right).

What you must avoid at all costs is having no plan or having a plan but spontaneously deviating from it when tempted. Traveling gives you continual opportunities to strengthen either your resistance muscle or your giving-in muscle; that's why continuing to plan your food intake in advance is so important.

You will need some strong responses to counteract sabotaging thoughts. Think back to trips in the past. Can you remember losing control of your eating and then feeling guilty and frustrated with yourself—if not while you were away, then when you came back and got on the scale? Or have you ever come back and avoided the scale for the next few days or weeks? Was it worth it? Some dieters report that they had done so well on diets until they traveled. Then they got off track and were unable to get themselves back on a diet for a very long time.

To travel successfully, you will probably need to repeatedly read many of the Response Cards from earlier in this chapter and this book. In addition, here is a special travel-oriented Response Card:

---

TRAVEL RESPONSE CARD

It's worth it to me to stay in control while I'm away.
The consequences of getting out of control are too
severe. If I cheat, it will put a damper on the trip.
I'll feel guilty and bad about myself. I'll be strengthening my giving-in muscle. If I stand firm, I can still
enjoy every bite of food I plan to have and I'll feel good
about myself both on the trip and when I return home.

---

# The Travel Calories Decision

Make an important rule for yourself, similar to the Special Event Calories decision. Be prepared before the next time you travel. You can opt to:

- Follow your Think Thin Eating Plan as is.

**OR**

- Eat up to 300 extra Travel Calories as often as every day you are away (for not more than a week and as long as you plan in advance how to use the extra calories).

There are advantages and disadvantages to either decision. Sticking to your regular plan makes life easier because you will have less opportunity to obsess over how to spend the extra calories and less planning to do, and you are more likely to lose—or at least maintain—weight while you are away. And you will still have daily Bonus Calories. But it may be difficult to maintain this rule the entire time you are gone. If you might eat too much, it's better to have an extra Travel Calories rule than to violate a No Travel Calories rule that could lead to more mistakes.

If you choose extra Travel Calories, you will have more choice of food and drink. But there are disadvantages. You will have to find out the calorie content of what you plan to have. More freedom puts you at risk for additional overeating and cravings while you are away. You may also have a difficult time getting back on track when you return and have to give up those extra calories. You will likely gain some weight (but once you return to normal eating, the weight will come off).

Decide what your rule will be. In your Diet Notebook under "Travel Plan," write either:

* *I am making the choice to follow my regular Think Thin Eating Plan.*

**OR**

* *My rule for traveling is:*
  *I can have up to _____ extra calories (fill in a number up to 300) on up to _____ days (fill in a number between 1 and 7). I can eat these extra calories only if I have planned to do so in advance. I can't use them spontaneously.*

Implement your chosen rule the next time you travel to see how well it works for you. Jordan found his rule to stick to his Think Thin Eating Plan too limiting, especially since he ate every meal for a week in restaurants. So he decided to eat 300 extra calories every other day of his six-day trip. The number on the scale went up a pound and a half. When he returned home, however, Jordan went back to his normal eating, continued to weigh himself, and lost the extra weight in the following week.

Nancy decided it wasn't worth using Travel Calories on subsequent trips because it had taken her so long to lose even the small amount of weight she had gained on a previous trip. When she travels, she continually reminds herself why it's worth it to stick to her usual number of calories. After practicing her new rule on several trips, it became much easier for Nancy to stick to her plan. She now has the confidence to do it, and her determination has grown because she knows it's worth it.

Once you figure out the best rule for you, I think you'll find it a big relief to have a plan that keeps you in control, minimizes weight gain, and leaves you feeling good about yourself throughout every trip you take in the future.

# travel skills

When you travel, you have less control over your food for a longer period of time than in practically any other situation. You will probably need to use all of your Challenging Situation Skills, as well as some additional ones listed below.

## Before You Go

**Pack your dieting supplies:** Bring this book, as well as your Response Cards, Advantages Deck, Cheat Sheet, and Diet Notebook. Consider bringing your food scale and measuring cups and spoons, if you will be eating in. Some dieters, who know they won't have the opportunity to buy their own food when they are away, like to bring snacks, such as nuts, canned tuna, cheese, fruits, or high-fiber/high-protein bars. Other dieters know it is better

**tip:** If you do eat unplanned food, don't use it as an excuse to continue eating unplanned food until your trip is over. Read your Cheat Sheet. Answer the questions and get back on track immediately. Don't compound the problem by continuing to eat more, because it's just not worth it. If you overeat at the beginning of the trip, you might gain a little weight. If you continue to overeat, you might gain a lot of weight. Which scenario would you prefer?

for them to make do with whatever food is available because carrying extra food is too tempting.

**On your way:** Read your Response Cards and relevant sections in your Diet Notebook on the trip there. If you haven't packed food to eat on the way, and the only available foods are relatively high in calories, you'll have to eat small portions. Remember, if you're still hungry, it's not an emergency! You will have another snack or meal coming up in a few hours or the following morning.

**Your arrival:** If you are staying in a hotel, the treats in your room can be very tempting. Put them in a closet, cover them with a towel, or ask the hotel staff to remove them. You can also give back the mini-bar key.

**During the trip:** You may have to use every Challenging Situation Skill from pages 131–164 to resist eating unplanned food. Read your Response Cards regularly. Get back on track immediately if you make a mistake, or you will likely find that your mood is adversely affected for the rest of the trip. It's worth it to stick with the plan, and it will get so much easier the more you practice.

**After the trip:** On the way home, plan your meals for the rest of the day and the next day. If you get on the scale and find you have gained weight, don't get discouraged! Reread pages 102–105 to get yourself back on track.

## Memory Box Cards

The first time you follow your plan while traveling and find that experience meaningful, file it in your Memory Box. Make subsequent cards for any future trips with meaningful experiences. This is what Renée wrote on a Memory Card:

---

### Memory Card

I usually *overeat* when I travel, but this time I packed lunch and a snack ahead of time. It felt really good to eat in a healthy way, and I felt much better than I usually do when I got to the hotel. I managed to skip all of the snacks from the mini-bar—I've never been able to do that before. Although I think the portions I took one night were too big, I basically stayed in control the whole time.

---

# Confidently Follow Your Plan When Life Gets Stressful

You've learned the skill of making time for dieting. But sometimes, no matter how well you practice this skill, life gets in the way: You have to fit in a series of dental appointments; you get in a fender bender and then lose the use of your car for a week; you strain your back; one of your parents is in the hospital; you take a second job.

A University of Toronto study shows that during harried times many people tend to comfort themselves with food, especially candy, chocolate, cakes, and chips. However, such life stressors don't have to be recipes for diet failure. You can follow your diet no matter what—if you're prepared.

## Create a Stressful Times Mindset

When people are stressed, they often give themselves permission to let things slip. They stop running errands, put off routine medical visits, call their friends or family less frequently. Dieters, in particular, get loose with eating and exercising. They fail to plan their meals in advance or go to the market often enough. They grab food on the run, eat unplanned food, and simply don't make time to exercise.

One common sabotaging thought they have is, *I deserve to comfort myself with food*. If you have that thought, agree with the first part of it but respond to the second part. Of course, it's true that you deserve comfort. But if you seek comfort in food, you will only end up feeling more stressed and out of control—and you may gain weight. Instead, do what successful maintainers do when they feel stressed. They look to other people for comfort. They treat themselves to something special, such as a massage. They pray or do meditation or yoga.

A second common thought is, *I just don't care anymore*. This statement is probably both true *and* false. You probably don't care as much at that moment. But you probably will care very much the next time you get on the scale or suffer other negative consequences of overeating. And even if you don't care very much that moment, try projecting ahead to when the stressful time is over. Will you care then?

A third thought is, *I can't do it anymore; dieting is too hard*. This thought usually arises when dieters have had intermittent difficulty practicing their skills for several days, but the experience of a few hours colors their memory of *entire* days or weeks. Whenever you feel burdened by life's stresses, ask yourself, *Has sticking to my diet been difficult for every hour of every day?* Or were there some hours or even days that it was easier? If you feel overburdened, identify the specific times or situations in which dieting was difficult. Ask your Diet Buddy for help in identifying times of trouble.

Prepare for such sabotaging thoughts by making Response Cards:

## UNDER STRESS REPONSE CARD #1

It's true I'm under a lot of stress right now. But sticking to my plan isn't hard every hour of every day. And, in fact, there are times when sticking to my plan has made life easier because I didn't have to think about or struggle over food. It's not worth it to me to throw in the towel and stop watching what I eat because I will definitely gain weight, feel bad about myself, and feel even more stressed.

## UNDER STRESS RESPONSE CARD #2

I will feel generally more in control if I control my eating. But I do need to look for other ways to comfort myself. Food is just a momentary distraction that comes with really negative consequences. When this stressful period ends, I know I won't want to be heavier.

# skills for when you are under stress

You will need most of the same skills as for other challenging situations:

- Review your Response Cards and Advantages Deck often.

- Use your Resistance Techniques.

- Check in with your Diet Buddy to stay accountable.

- Imagine the aftermath (gaining weight once this stressful period ends versus maintaining or losing weight).

- Use your Cheat Sheet.

- Weigh yourself every morning.

In addition, you can decide whether you want to stay at your current calorie level or go up to the next level for a predetermined period of time. It may be reasonable to add a little more food (especially if you have less control over your food), even if you stay the same weight or gain a little.

You may also need to do some problem solving to reduce your stress. Ask yourself the following questions:

- *What do I need help with?*

- *Whom can I ask for help?*

- *Which self-care activities am I neglecting?*

- *Which tasks, responsibilities, or activities do I temporarily need to postpone, do less of, do less well, or delegate to others?*

- *Would anyone be as stressed in this situation as I am? If my negative reaction is greater than other people's reaction would be, maybe I need help to put things in better perspective.*

## Special Advice for When You Are Sick or Injured

Many dieters get completely derailed when they are indisposed. They view their situation in an all-or-nothing way: *Because I'm ailing, I can't follow my diet at all,* or, *Because I can't do my usual exercise, it's not worth doing any.* They frequently go back to old habits, gain weight, and have difficulty reestablishing their diet and exercise programs once they are well. They have many of the sabotaging thoughts described in the previous section, and the same Response Cards and skills apply.

On the other hand, when dieters are sick, they often don't want to eat as much as usual, and they have the sabotaging thought, *I should take advantage of the fact that my appetite is reduced to eat as few calories as possible.* This is usually counter-productive to their recovery, and they often regain any weight they had lost—if not more—as soon as they are feeling better and eating normally again. Resist the temptation to eat in an unhealthy way when you're under the weather.

Even when you are sick or injured, stay as close as possible to your diet and exercise programs. If you can't do your regular exercise, check with your health-care provider to see what you *can* do. Maybe you can swim or work out on machines that strengthen the uninjured parts of your body. Consider whether it would be helpful to consult with a physical therapist. And when you recover, make sure to build up to your previous level of exercise as slowly as you need to.

## Before You Move On

In the next stage, you will learn how to implement a more flexible way of eating. Many dieters want to jump the gun and start this new stage too soon. Don't be fooled! It is essential to have mastered inflexible eating skills first. At some point, you will find that instead of becoming flexible, your eating has become too loose. You may also become lax in your eating habits. And your weight will start to go up. At that point, you should return to inflexible eating until your weight comes back down.

However, if you never mastered inflexible eating in the first place, you may have a very tough time getting back in control and losing weight. I bet that has happened to you in the past and prevented you from achieving lasting weight loss up to this point. But mastering all of the skills in Stages 1–3 will ensure that this never has to happen ever again because you will always know exactly what to do!

As you work on your Stage 3 skills, don't forget to keep adding more movement to your day. Continue to increase your planned exercise, including cardiovascular and strength training.

You will know that you are ready for Stage 4 when you have faithfully followed your Think Thin Initial Eating Plan and have implemented your Stages 1, 2, and 3 Success Skills consistently for a few weeks in a row. You will also have changed your basic attitude toward food and eating. You will have gone from, *This is so hard ... This requires so much effort,* to, *This is pretty easy most of the time ... And even when it's more difficult, it's so worth it to me to stay in control.*

Remain in Stage 3 until you've made that shift:

| From Automatically Thinking This: | to | Thinking This: |
|---|---|---|
| *Dieting is so hard.* | ⟶ | *I know I can keep this up.* |
| *I wish I didn't have to exercise.* | ⟶ | *I feel good when I exercise.* |
| *It's unfair that I can't eat like everyone else.* | ⟶ | *This is how all successful dieters and maintainers eat.* |
| *I messed up. I might as well give up and eat whatever I want.* | ⟶ | *I made a mistake. It won't even show up on the scale if I get back on track now.* |
| *I wish I could have eaten more.* | ⟶ | *I'm so glad I followed my plan.* |
| *What if I get hungry?* | ⟶ | *Hunger isn't a big deal. I'll eat again in a few hours or tomorrow morning.* |
| *It's rude to turn down food.* | ⟶ | *It's important for me to stick up for myself.* |
| *I should be able to treat myself in special situations.* | ⟶ | *I can eat what I want as long as I plan in advance to use my Bonus Calories for it.* |
| *When I'm stressed I need to eat.* | ⟶ | *I can deal with stressful situations without turning to food. And I'm always so glad when I do.* |

Once you've made these important thinking shifts, you are ready for Stage 4: The Think Thin Lifetime Eating Plan.

# chapter 7

# Stage 4

## The Think Thin Lifetime Eating Plan

Once you have learned to follow your plan in any situation, you are probably ready to learn how to be more flexible with your eating—if the following statements are true:

- You are committed to keep practicing all of your Success Skills and to solve any problems that arise in implementing them every day.

- You know, without question, that you can tolerate hunger and cravings.

- You can have tempting food right in front of you and confidently tell yourself, *No, I didn't plan to eat it, so I'm not going to have any.*

- You can enjoy reasonable amounts of any food without losing control.

If you meet these criteria, congratulations! You now have the self-control to start varying what (and perhaps when) you eat. If, on the other hand, you haven't yet mastered the skills you need, don't worry. Go back and reread the first three stages; then do every task again. It takes dieters varying amounts of time to fully master the skills in these stages, so make sure you go as slowly as you need to.

Even if you have met all of the prerequisites, you don't have to transition to flexible eating now. Are you having such thoughts as, *I'm losing weight ... I don't want to rock the boat!* That's okay—you don't have to start right away. Mark your calendar to revisit your decision in a month or so to see if you feel ready then.

It's important to make this transition at some point because you never know when life will throw you a diet-related curveball. Inevitably something unexpected will happen. Maybe you will start a new relationship, begin caring for a sick relative, or work new hours. Flexible eating will teach you how to stick with your diet by creating an alternative plan. It's important for you to prove to yourself that you can eat more flexibly and still lose weight—and keep it off. Remember, flexible eating is a skill like everything else. It takes practice, and it gets easier over time.

As you make this transition, remain inflexible about checking off your skills every night on your Stage 4 Success Skills Sheet (pages 272–273). To guard against falling back into unhelpful habits, you will need the Success Skills Sheet to remind you what you need to do—and to keep yourself honest. Old habits sometimes die hard; you will need to stay vigilant. Continue to increase your spontaneous exercise; in addition, work up to a minimum of 30 minutes of daily movement and twice-weekly strength training.

In this chapter, you will:

- Conduct experiments to choose variations of the Think Thin Eating Plan.

- Create a customized Think Thin Lifetime Eating Plan.

- Modify your Think Thin Lifetime Eating Plan when you plateau, move into maintenance, or encounter changing life circumstances.

## Experiments to Vary the Think Thin Eating Plan

You will do experiments to decide whether—and how—you want to vary the number and timing of your snacks, as well as the foods you eat for snacks and meals. You will use the results of these experiments to build variations into the Think Thin Initial Eating Plan to create a customized Think Thin Lifetime Eating Plan.

I didn't want you to do these experiments in an earlier stage because I wanted to make sure your hunger was minimized as you learned how to stick to your food plan. I also wanted you to experience for many weeks the wonderful benefits of healthful eating. And I wanted you to have the chance to enjoy simple, healthful, unprocessed food. Have you found, as many dieters have, that your taste buds have actually changed? Many find that they just don't enjoy high-fat or refined foods nearly as much and don't feel as well after eating them. Other dieters find it just isn't worth eating foods that lead them to experience more cravings.

In your Diet Notebook, create a page titled "Think Thin Lifetime Eating Plan."

Try any or all of the experiments below. If an experiment works well and you want to continue implementing that particular variation, write it down under the subtitle "Optional Guidelines." Note that at this point, you will need to plan in advance to continue doing the variation described in the experiment. In the final steps of this stage, you will be able to make changes in the moment. There are six experiments; the first three do not entail counting calories, but the second three do:

1. Add your snack foods to meals.

2. Change the timing of your snacks.

3. Swap one Think Thin Eating Plan meal for another.

4. Trade Think Thin Initial Eating Plan foods with equal-calorie foods.

5. Add snack calories to the next meal.

6. Bank all snack calories for a special meal.

# experiment 1

## Add your snack foods to meals.

Some dieters prefer to have larger meals instead of snacks. You can do an experiment to see if this works well for you. Take the food you would have eaten for a snack (from Snack Options, page 224) and add it to another meal. You can add your midmorning snack to breakfast or to lunch, your midafternoon snack to lunch or to dinner, and/or your evening snack to dinner. Find out:

• Do you like having a larger meal instead of a snack?

• Do you get overly hungry between meals?

• Does skipping snacks set up cravings for unplanned food?

While some dieters can easily skip a snack, others can't. For example, Jane decided to forgo her afternoon snack so she could add her snack food to dinner. But then she found herself nibbling on food—standing up—as she prepared dinner because she was hungry after skipping her usual snack.

If adding your snack food to meals works well for you, you can opt to make it part of your Think Thin Lifetime Eating Plan. Write it down in your Diet Notebook under "Optional Guidelines." For example, you might write, "Add morning snack to breakfast; choose from Snack Options." At this point, you will plan in advance to make this change. A later step will be to decide whether to have a snack in the moment.

# experiment 2

## Change the timing of your snacks.

Some dieters have the most difficulty sticking to their plans in the evening. If you like, try skipping your morning or afternoon snack and have two snacks in the evening instead of one. (Or you could try splitting your evening snack in two and then eat the food at two different times.) Or if you eat dinner late, try skipping your evening snack and having two afternoon snacks. If either variation works well, record it in your Diet Notebook. You might write, "Have a snack at midmorning, 3 p.m., and 6 p.m. Skip after-dinner snack. Choose from Snack Options."

# experiment 3

## Swap one Think Thin Eating Plan meal for another.

There are two additional ways you can easily customize your Think Thin Lifetime Eating Plan that don't entail figuring out calories. You can:

- Switch your Think Thin meals. For example, have your dinner options at lunchtime and your lunch options at dinnertime. See if you prefer having a larger lunch and smaller dinner.

- Use the recipes on pages 230–262. These contain the appropriate number of calories for each meal, and I think you'll enjoy the variety.

If any of these experiments work out well, you can build these optional variations into your Think Thin Lifetime Eating Plan. Write them in your Diet Notebook under "Optional Guidelines" and plan in advance when you are going to implement them.

The rest of the experiments entail choosing a greater variety of food than the Think Thin Initial Eating Plan contains. To conduct these experiments, you will have to figure out calorie contents by reading labels or using the lists in Chapter 10, a calorie book, or such online resources as the one listed on page 264.

Here is how to read a food-package label without getting fooled: Look at the box with the nutrition information. Note both the number of calories listed and the serving size. Many packaged foods may seem as if they contain just one serving, but they actually contain more. For example, I recently looked at the nutrition facts label for a packaged cookie at a coffee shop. It said, "190 calories per serving." When I looked to see how many servings the cookie contained, it wasn't one—it was two and a half. The entire cookie was 475 calories!

## Discover How Marketers Try to Get You to Buy

The food industry spends $36 billion annually in an effort to get you to buy specific products. Packaging frequently contains misleading stages that many consumer advocates call "nutri-washing." These nutri-washing phrases make many relatively unhealthful foods seem healthful. These phrases include:

• **"Made with whole grain."** If the majority of the ingredients listed on the label are sugar, corn oil, cornstarch, corn syrup, dextrose, dyes, and artificial colors and flavors, then the few whole grains contained in the product can do little to make this product a healthful choice.

• **"All-natural."** There is no government guideline for this claim, so any product can proclaim to be all natural, even if every ingredient is processed.

• **"Trans fat–free."** Products with this claim are allowed by law to contain small amounts of this unhealthy fat—but many health experts believe that *any* amount of trans fat above zero is too much. Always check the list of ingredients for the word *hydrogenated*. If you see that word, the product contains trans fat, despite product advertising.

• **"Calorie-free," "light," "reduced-calorie," or "sugar-free."** Foods with these tags may still contain a considerable amount of calories. Government regulations, for example, allow "calorie-free" foods, such as packets of artificial sweeteners, to contain up to 5 calories per serving. "Low-calorie" foods may contain up to 40 calories per serving. "Reduced-calorie" and "lower-in-calorie" foods only need to have 25 percent fewer calories than their higher-calorie versions— and for "light" foods, a third of the calories as their regular counterparts. Some "sugar-free" foods are still quite caloric. Check the calorie amounts on the nutrition facts label to determine for yourself whether they fit into the calorie count for your snack or meal.

• **"Reduced-fat."** Not all reduced-fat foods are reduced in calories, too. Some replace the fat with sugar or other types of carbohydrate. For example, reduced-fat peanut butter usually contains the same number of calories as the full-fat version due to the addition of extra sugar.

# experiment 4

## Trade Think Thin Initial Eating Plan foods with equal-calorie foods.

If you would like to occasionally include a favorite less-healthful food in place of a Think Thin Eating Plan food, you will need to do some experiments. Be sure to keep the number of calories the same within each swap, but—be forewarned—the portion size you are allowed will probably shrink.

For example, in the experiments below, you will be able to trade food and see what happens to your levels of hunger, cravings, and energy if you:

- Swap a sugar-sweetened cereal for your usual breakfast selection.

- Skip eating protein; have a salad and pasta with marinara sauce at lunch or dinner.

- Choose white bread instead of whole-wheat bread.

- Have a small piece of fried chicken (or chicken with a special sauce) in place of a larger piece of grilled chicken.

Plan in advance to make the trade and stay within your calorie limits both for that part of the meal and for the meal as a whole. At most, change just one food a day to help you pinpoint how each change is affecting you.

**If you notice no difference in your hunger, cravings, or desire to eat,** then go ahead and add these foods to your Think Thin Lifetime Eating Plan if you wish. In your Diet Notebook, write, "Trade Think Thin foods for same-calorie foods as often as desired if foods are healthful; no more than once a week if foods are not." The foods you eat should be as healthful as possible to reduce your risk of heart disease, cancer, diabetes, and other medical problems.

**If you notice that you feel hungrier between meals,** finish what is on your plate and want more, have an increased desire to eat other foods that are not on your plan, or feel a little unwell after eating, you may decide it isn't worth it to incorporate these changes. If you want to continue to include a particular new food in your repertoire, you may have to work harder to cope with hunger, cravings, and desire.

# experiment 5

### Add snack calories to the next meal.

You can plan in advance to skip a snack and use the snack *calories* (not necessarily a snack from the Snack Options) to add any kind of food with the same number of calories to your next meal. This means you can have an extra side dish, a larger portion, or additional ingredients in your dishes. Maybe you would like to have a dinner roll, eat extra steak, or put a special sauce on your vegetables without using your Bonus Calories. Of course, this means that you will have to calculate in advance how much of the extra food you can have. If you would like to continue doing this, write in your Diet Notebook, "Add snack calories to the next meal as often as desired if food is healthful; up to once a week if food is not particularly healthful."

# experiment 6

## Bank all snack calories for a special meal.

You can also decide in advance to *occasionally* pool the calories from all three snacks and add them to one meal. For example, you might choose one of the following:

- An appetizer and/or bread

- A mixed drink or more than one glass of wine or beer

- A special higher-calorie dish

- A larger portion of one or more foods

- A full-sized serving of dessert

Make sure to look up the calorie count of any food or drink you want to have. Don't get fooled. You may find that many foods and beverages have far more calories than you expect. For example:

- One 6-ounce glass of wine totals about 150 calories, a light 12-ounce beer totals 100 calories, and a regular 12-ounce beer has 150 calories.

- Mixed drinks range from about 200 to 400 calories.

- Specialty coffee drinks range from 120 or more calories for a small nonfat latte to over 400 calories for other sugar- and cream-laden drinks.

- Appetizers typically served on party platters range from 40 to 250 calories per piece.

- Many fried appetizers served at restaurants are meals in themselves. A deep-fried eggroll may contain 200 calories, fried calamari may total 350 to 700 calories, onion rings may have 300 to 700 calories, and buffalo wings may be 50 to 100 calories each.

- A 12-ounce New York strip steak equals about 750 calories.

- One slice of cheesecake, pie, or homemade chocolate cake with frosting may have 250 to 400 calories; double those amounts for larger restaurant portions.

Don't make the mistake of estimating on the low side, or you'll be unhappy when you step on the scale. Plan in advance to try this experiment and keep tabs on your hunger, cravings, and ability to stay in control. Some dieters can easily stick to their plans. But others can't. When Doug skipped his snacks, he later not only ordered an appetizer (planned), but also he had a full-sized dessert that he did not split with anyone (unplanned). If you make this kind of mistake, you may not yet be ready for this approach.

If you would like, write this variation in your Diet Notebook, adding, "Not more than once a week." I don't want you to get into the habit of spending snack calories on less-healthy food or having much-larger-than-usual portions. Kris made a rule for herself that she would bank calories only once a month because she finds that even though she is careful, she has a tendency to go beyond the allotted number of calories, particularly if she spends them on alcohol or dessert. She marks on a calendar whenever she banks them so she doesn't forget that she has done so.

Now that you have tried these experiments, it is time to make a customized Think Thin Lifetime Eating Plan. In the sections below, you will:

- Create your own recipes and meals.

- Learn to change your plan in the moment.

- Stay flexible but in control.

- Develop a general plan.

- Mentally plan your week.

## Create Your Own Recipes and Meals

You no longer have to be limited by the foods listed in this book. You can create your personal repertoire of recipes and meals for your Think Thin Lifetime Eating Plan. To do so, stick with the calorie level for each component of a meal (protein, whole grain, vegetable, etc.) and for the meal as a whole. Follow the food lists (pages 215–227) as a guide and use a calorie counter to ensure you consume the right number of calories. You can also use a number of convenient online tools to help you determine the calories per serving in your favorite recipes. I've included a sample Web site in Chapter 12 (page 264).

For example, Nina really loved veal parmigiana, so she decided to convert it to a Think Thin Lifetime Eating Plan dish. She looked up the calorie amounts for all of the ingredients she used to make her favorite recipe. She discovered that the lean veal she used contained 35 calories per ounce, the breadcrumbs 200 calories per ½ cup, the sauce 150 calories per cup, and the cheese 160 calories per half cup. She decided to bake the veal rather than fry it to save calories. Once she crunched the numbers, she determined that all of her ingredients for the dish totaled 1,000 calories. She divided that by 4 to create a portion that corresponded to the calorie plan she was following. She enjoyed her low-calorie portion with a side salad with squeezed lemon, steamed broccoli and cauliflower, and a small whole-wheat dinner roll dipped in 1 teaspoon of olive oil.

In addition to making sure each dish conforms to the calorie guidelines of the plan you are using, also do the following to maximize satiation and health:

**Make each meal balanced.** Include reasonable amounts of protein, vegetables, and whole grains at every lunch and dinner. Roughly half of your lunch or dinner plate should be taken up with vegetables. On the other half, roughly two-thirds should be protein and the rest grains.

**Keep protein lean.** Choose extra-lean red meat, skinless poultry, pork, fish, or seafood, for example, so you can serve yourself larger portions.

**Choose whole grains.** They contain more nutrients and fiber than refined grains, which have been stripped of their outer hulls and germ. The fiber makes them more filling for the same number of calories. Select brown or wild rice instead of white; whole-grain bread instead of refined; and potatoes with the skin on to maximize nutrients and the filling effects of whole-grain fiber.

**Keep fats healthy.** Primarily choose such non-saturated fats as olive oil, trans fat–free margarine, fish, olives, nuts, seeds, and avocados. Avoid trans fat (found in processed foods and fried foods) and saturated fats (found in fatty animal products). Both can raise your risk of heart disease and cancer.

**Choose packaged foods that are as high in protein and fiber and as low in sugar as possible.** But avoid packaged foods when possible to minimize your intake of unhealthy additives.

**Create a new subtitle, "Recipes and Menus,"** in your Diet Notebook on your Think Thin Lifetime Eating Plan page. Organize this section in any way that you wish. You might include subsections for breakfast, lunch, dinner, and snacks. When you write down a recipe, include the measurement of each ingredient to make sure you stay within your calorie limits every time you make it. Keep adding to this section as you create more and more customized dishes.

## Learn to Change Your Plan in the Moment

Until now you have followed your plan precisely, and if you've fully mastered the skill of sticking to it and staying in control, you're probably ready to learn how to change it in the moment. Let's say you planned to have the turkey sandwich you packed for lunch, but a coworker offers pizza. Before this point, you had to turn down your coworker because you hadn't planned in advance to have pizza. If you really wanted it, you would have had to wait until the next day. Now, you can experiment:

- You can make your snacks optional and decide at the last minute whether to have one or add it to a later meal.

- You can change your mind and eat something you haven't planned as long as:

  - It is at a planned snack time or mealtime. (Otherwise, you'll be strengthening your giving-in muscle.)

  - You stay within the calorie limit for that snack or meal.

  - You maintain the nutritional balance of the snack or meal (including the appropriate balance of protein, grains, vegetables, and fat).

Whenever you alter your plan spontaneously, pay careful attention to whether you are doing it for a legitimate reason:

- It's not legitimate to skip the protein, vegetables, and grain you planned for dinner and have ice cream instead.

- It's not legitimate to change your plan because you're eating for emotional reasons.

- It's not legitimate to skimp on one meal so you can eat more at another.

- It's not legitimate to break a rule. If you are like I am and have the rule, *I will never eat sweets at work,* don't break the rule at the last minute just because the brownies in the office kitchen look really good. You can re-examine your rule the next day, when you're feeling calm and satisfied and then change it if you want. (For example, you might decide that it's okay to use your Bonus Calories at work one day a week instead of saving them for another time in the day.)

If you find that you are continually adjusting your plan, you may need to do some problem solving:

- Have you been craving more?

- Have you been too tired to cook?

- Have you been too rushed to prepare the food you had planned?

- Have you neglected to go to the market for the food you need?

- Have you stopped making some of your meals for the week during the weekend?

If so, solve these problems now so they don't continually crop up. If you don't, you will run into trouble sooner or later. You may need to reread pages 41–42 to re-prioritize dieting.

Again, all of these are just experiments for you to try (if you wish). If you find that any of them make you struggle more often or make it generally harder to stick to your diet, it's probably better for you to forgo that particular variation. Although it gets so much easier, dieting can still be difficult from time to time, and it's worth doing everything you can to make it as easy and painless as possible.

## Stay Flexible but in Control

Flexible eating is challenging, especially in the beginning. You have to figure out whether a last-minute modification is legitimate (for example, you substitute one healthful meal for another) or not (you give in to a craving and have an unscheduled snack). You may find, as you get more flexible with your eating, that you become too loose.

Dennis had been doing very well on the Beck Diet for Life Program. He had lost 45 pounds. But he gradually ran into trouble. One day he altered his usual plan of consuming his Bonus Calories for an evening snack. He wanted a larger evening treat and made up for it by having a smaller dinner (a violation of the guidelines). He liked doing this and gradually started doing it more often. At first he easily stayed within his calorie limits, and the number on the scale didn't go up. After doing this on and off for a couple of weeks, he drifted back into eating his normal dinner and a larger evening snack because the higher-calorie snack had psychologically become his new "normal."

Dennis got away with the extra calories for a few days, but in less than a week, his weight started to slowly increase. When he realized what was going on, Dennis quickly went back to having just his planned Bonus Calories in the evenings, and he was able to shed the added weight. Like Dennis, many dieters initially struggle somewhat with flexible eating, but the more they work at it, the easier and more natural it becomes.

What's the difference between flexible eating and loose eating? Consult the chart below:

| Flexible Eating, Not Loose Eating | |
| --- | --- |
| **Flexible Eating** | **Loose Eating** |
| Making a conscious choice to adjust your plan, counting every calorie and staying with preset limits | Changing your plan and ignoring the calorie count or nutritional content |
| Skipping your morning, afternoon, or evening snack so that you can eat a larger-than-usual dinner | Eating a larger dinner without reducing your snack calories |
| Making a conscious decision to eat on the run because something unexpected came up | Eating a rushed meal on the go because you stopped making time for dieting |

What are other indications that you are getting too loose?

- **You have stopped practicing your skills regularly.** Whether or not you're eating flexibly, you still need to practice all of your skills and to fill in your Stage 4 Success Skills Sheet (pages 272–273) every night. Are you eating all of your food slowly, while sitting down and enjoying every bite? Or have you lapsed into tasting unplanned food from your dining companion's plate or sneaking bites as you clear the table? Are you giving yourself credit? Are you still reading your Response Cards and Advantages Deck? Reading them every morning—and at vulnerable times of the day—is crucial at this stage. With more choices, you may begin to struggle again. I want you to be completely conscious at all times why it's so important—and so worth it—to stay in control. If you find that you're slipping, go back to Stage 1 and make a concerted effort to use every skill as you adjust to flexible eating. Then if you still experience difficulty, go back to the Think Thin Initial Eating Plan in Stage 2 until you have firmly re-established your skills. Continue checking in with your Diet Buddy.

- **You have stopped weighing and measuring food altogether.** You may not have to weigh and measure every time, but you should continue to do so occasionally to make sure you are serving yourself the correct portions (and also when you introduce a new food into your diet). I've found that once dieters completely stop weighing and measuring their food, their portions tend to grow larger. A ½-cup serving of ice cream can slowly become ¾ cup—and then even a whole cup.

You can probably get away with being looser with your eating for a few days without ill effects showing up on the scale, but I can promise you that eating too many calories will catch up with you soon. It always does. That's why you will continue to weigh yourself every morning—to catch looseness before it turns into extra pounds.

## Develop a General Plan

You have decided whether to stick with three meals and three snacks a day, add snack food to other meals, or make snacks optional. You have figured out which menu choices work best for you and created customized meals based on the Think Thin Formula. Now, it's time to write a general plan in your Diet Notebook. You will follow this plan most of the time, only occasionally making permitted exceptions, as described earlier in this chapter.

Ginny recognized that she managed best when she added her midmorning snack to lunch and then used Bonus Calories for a second evening snack. She found it easiest to stick to the meals provided in the book for breakfast and lunch. She added a few high-protein snacks and customized some of her dinners, based on her own recipes, all of which she had already recorded in her Diet Notebook. Based on her current calorie level, Ginny wrote the plan on page 180 in her notebook.

Over time, Ginny found that she tended to eat many of the same foods day after day. Ginny could have potentially created countless different meals using the Think Thin guidelines, but she discovered which foods and meals she liked best, were most convenient to prepare, and kept her feeling full and satisfied. She usually chose from among three breakfasts, five lunches, and 10 dinners. Sometimes she alternated breakfasts each morning, and sometimes she selected the same breakfast for weeks at a time before switching off to another one. Ginny tended to do the same with her Bonus Calories. She alternated lunches and snacks more often, and dinners were the most variable (page 180).

**tip:** It's okay to occasionally eat on the run or standing up when you have a legitimate reason to do so. If you are at a party and there is no place to sit down, it's now okay to eat while standing, if you make a strong effort to enjoy every bite. If you are unusually rushed, it's okay to grab a meal on the go. Make sure these variations remain exceptions and not the norm.

> My Think Thin Eating Plan
>
> **Breakfast:** Any breakfast from page 215 or breakfast recipe from pages 230–232
>
> **Lunch:** Any lunch from pages 216–217 or lunch recipe from pages 234–236 and 256–258
>
> **Midafternoon Snack:** Any snack from page 224 or snack recipe from pages 251–255
>
> **Dinner:** Any dinner from page 218 or dinner recipe from pages 237–247 and 259–262 or from my list
>
> **Evening Snack #1:** Any snack from page 224 or snack recipe from pages 251–255 or from my list
>
> **Evening Snack #2:** 150 Bonus Calories of whatever I want

When they first come to see me, many dieters initially resist the idea of limiting their breakfast and lunch choices. They believe they will always want to have a large variety of foods. I tell them that's fine; in fact, I want them to try as many different options as possible. But I almost always find that down the line, they just naturally end up eating a limited variety of foods because they discover, as Ginny did, that having fewer choices makes their lives easier and they now know which foods really work best for them.

## Mentally Plan Your Week

Once you master the art of flexible eating and you have a workable general plan, you no longer have to write down in advance what you plan to eat (although you are welcome to continue doing so if you wish). You can experiment with mental planning. If you find that you are making too many spontaneous decisions, eating too many calories for some meals or snacks, obsessing about what to eat, or being too tempted by food, go back to putting your plan in writing and monitoring it as you go along. Return to mental planning at a later date.

Here's how to implement mental planning. Every week, look at the coming days and ask yourself the following questions:

- *Which meals will I make this week? Which groceries do I need to buy, and when will I buy them?*

- *Will I be rushed any day? Do I need to make meals in advance for that day?*

- *Will my schedule be irregular on any day? Should I change the timing of my snacks for that day?*

- *What food preparation or cooking do I need to do on the weekend so that I will have an easier time during the week?*

- *Do I have any special events coming up this week? Do I want to use Special Event Calories (pages 129–130) for one meal? Or do I want to make sure to save my Bonus Calories for that meal?*

- *Will I have any friends or relatives visiting this week, which may make it harder to stick to my plan (and therefore require more advance planning)?*

Every evening, look ahead to the next day. Make a mental plan by asking yourself these questions:

- *What will I eat for each meal and snack tomorrow?*

- *Which foods will I need, and do I have them on hand? If not, when will I get them?*

- *What preparation do I need to do, and when will I do it?*

- *Which potential obstacles could throw me off course?*

- *Which tempting situations might I find myself in?*

At some point, you will start asking yourself these questions automatically. Until then, copy these questions in your Diet Notebook under the heading "Mental Planning" and make sure to read them regularly.

✳✳✳✳✳✳✳✳✳✳✳✳✳

In this final section, you will be preparing for rest-of-your-life eating. You will learn how and when to alter your Think Thin Lifetime Eating Plan, determine at which point you should finalize your plan and move into maintenance, and decide what to do when your lifestyle or physiology changes.

## Change Your General Plan

You may need to modify your general plan when certain life circumstances arise or when your weight plateaus. Use these guidelines:

If your life changes, you may find that you need to vary the timing of your snacks or meals, or even the number of snacks you have. You may also find that you can't easily sustain your current calorie level. For example, maybe you have gone back to school, taken a new job, improved your social life, or had a child. It is perfectly reasonable to make the decision to step up to the next higher-calorie level and gain a few pounds. Just don't let yourself slip into eating more. Make sure to keep following your general plan every day. You can stay at your new calorie level indefinitely, or you can experiment with dropping back a level whenever you like.

When your weight plateaus, you should sit tight for several weeks and see what happens. Some people start to lose weight again, even when they keep their calorie and exercise levels constant. If your weight doesn't budge, go back to measuring your food and counting every calorie to make sure you're not underestimating your intake. If you have been calculating correctly, you can move down to the next lower-calorie level *if you are not already at 1,600 calories and if you think you can sustain this reduction indefinitely.* If you are already at 1,600 calories and need to lose more weight because you have a health problem, please arrange for a professional consultation to find out how to safely and nutritiously eat 1,400 calories a day.

## Decide When to Move into Maintenance

You will know you are ready for maintenance when:

- You reach your goal weight.

OR

- You get to the 1,600-calorie level and (barring a health problem) your weight plateaus for a long time.

OR

- You get to one of the higher-calorie levels, your weight plateaus, and you don't want to cut your calories or increase your exercise; or you don't think you can sustain a lower-calorie intake for the long term.

Many dieters never get to the 1,600-calorie level. They decide that the challenges involved with further restricting their eating are not worth the small amount of additional weight they might lose.

Patti had reduced her weight to 155 pounds. She plateaued at the 2,000-calorie level and had remained there for several months. Although she wanted to lose more weight, she decided it wasn't worth it to further restrict her eating. She had already lost 38 pounds, and she felt great. She had already experienced so many advantages of weight loss. She couldn't think of any real advantages she would reap if she lost another 5 pounds or so, but she could think of numerous disadvantages to restricting her eating below 2,000 calories. She decided to move on and enjoy the rest of her life.

The point at which the effort to stay at a certain calorie level outweighs the benefits is different for each dieter. Draw your line at a calorie level that you can see yourself sustaining for years.

## Accepting Your Maintenance Weight

If you are not at your "dream" weight, you may be greatly disappointed. If you had always hoped to be thinner, it can be quite a blow to find out that you should not even try to get to a lower weight, much less sustain that weight. It means your dream just isn't—and probably never was—realistic.

What might you suggest to your best friend if he/she were in this exact situation? Would you offer the following advice?

- **Be proud of yourself.** Just because you didn't get down to the weight you wanted to be doesn't mean you failed. You've succeeded. You've lost weight! That's an important accomplishment that many people never achieve. You're probably much healthier now, too.

- **Consider the relative unimportance of your weight.** Think about it. Your weight is really so superficial. You have so many more important, wonderful attributes. List what they are.

- **Put your weight in perspective.** Look at the other positives in your life. Give yourself credit for all of your other accomplishments in life. List them, too.

- **Improve your life in other ways.** Do all of the things you had put off doing until you lost excess weight.

In short, you wouldn't want your friend to dwell on his/her disappointment. You would want your friend to change to a healthier focus.

This is one of those very big "Oh, well" life situations: *Oh, well, I had always hoped I would be thinner … But I can't change my biology, so I may as well not struggle over it … I may as well accept it and go live my life.* And even though you may not become as slim as you had always hoped, I will bet that you have still achieved most of the items in your Advantages Deck and that your life and health are greatly improved. Don't forget about how much better things are now!

Even if you can't sustain a lower weight, you can still change your appearance if you want to. Buy new clothes. Experiment with hairstyles and makeup. Improve your posture. Smile more.

If you find your disappointment lingers and starts coloring your experience, you can write about it in a journal. Or some people find it helpful to talk to their Diet Buddy or a sympathetic friend or family member. Tell him/her you don't want help in problem solving, though. You just want to be able to express your disappointment aloud and get emotional support.

## Staying Within a 5-pound Weight Range

Once you reach your maintenance weight, start graphing your weight differently. No one stays at one set number every day. Most maintainers fluctuate by a few pounds from day to day. To remember that these small fluctuations are normal and temporary, draw a red horizontal line all the way across the graph at "Base Weight," which will now stand for your initial maintenance weight, and another line at 5 pounds heavier. Every day, plot your weight, and give yourself credit for staying between the two lines. If you drift up toward the top of your weight range for more than a week, check your eating habits and make sure you haven't gotten too loose.

## Raising Your Maintenance Range

Keep in mind that you might decide to raise your maintenance weight at some point. This will probably happen for one of three reasons:

**1. Your metabolism has slowed or your physiology is different.** If your metabolism changes—due to age, a medical condition, menopause, or a medication—you may decide to remain at your current calorie level and allow yourself to gain a few pounds.

**2. You have made a reasonable decision to exercise less.** You are still exercising enough to be healthy, but you don't have the time right now to do extra exercise; or perhaps an injury has limited your exercise capabilities.

**3. You want to have more calories to spend.** Perhaps you want to eat out more or indulge in an extra glass of wine several evenings a week. I want you to have a wonderful life! Of course, I want you to stay in control of your eating and weight, but I don't want you to stay so focused on the number on the scale and your daily calorie allotment that you miss out on getting as much enjoyment as you can. If the extra calories are worth it to you, then have them! It's fine to decide to eat more as long as you consciously make the decision to do so and haven't gotten loose with your eating. Just make sure that you continue to use good eating habits and get appropriate nutrition. Consider adding up to 200 more calories to your daily allotment (knowing that you may gain a few pounds), either temporarily or permanently. This is a legitimate change to your plan.

## Before You Move On

Keep increasing your exercise, filling out your Stage 4 Success Skills Sheet, contacting your Diet Buddy, and adding to your Advantages Deck and Memory Box.

I would like you to proceed to Stage 5 right away. But be alert for times when you may need to reread Stage 4. You may want to try additional experiments, assess whether you are slipping into loose eating, change your general plan, or decide if you should declare yourself in maintenance. Use Stage 4, as needed, for the rest of your life to ensure that you enjoy all of the benefits of flexible eating.

# chapter 8

# Stage 5

## The Motivation-for-Life Plan

Y ou've made it to Stage 5! My guess is that your mindset about food and dieting are completely different from before you started the Beck Diet for Life Program. You no longer fear hunger, cravings, or strong negative emotions. You know how to handle even the most challenging eating situations: restaurants, buffets, social gatherings, and much more. You know how to get yourself to do things you don't necessarily feel like doing because you know it's worth it. And you have also transitioned to an eating plan that you can comfortably follow for life because it allows you to create your own healthy recipes and meals and to make modifications as needed.

What else do you need to guarantee long-term success? A lifetime motivation plan. If you are like most dieters, you may find it difficult to believe that your motivation could ever flag—but at some point it will, even if you practice all of your skills consistently. It's just human nature to be accustomed to the status quo.

Dieters' motivation usually decreases when the rate at which they are losing weight has slowed or when they are in maintenance. In either case, they find that it's not as rewarding to step on the scale each morning because the number doesn't change very much. By this time, dieters may not feel the same degree of pleasure as they previously did, because it's no longer a new experience when they look in the mirror or shop for clothes. They also may not get as many compliments because the

**Healthful eating will probably always take some effort, but it generally gets easier as time goes on. If you don't put in the effort, you will lose the advantages you have gained. Isn't it worth it to keep making the effort?**

people around them have also become accustomed to their weight loss. On a day-to-day basis, most dieters get so used to living with their thinner, healthier bodies that they don't even think very much about how they looked when they were heavier; had to wear larger-sized clothing; felt embarrassed or self-conscious in many situations; were less energetic and less healthy; and generally just didn't feel very good about themselves.

Like most dieters, it is likely that you will eventually begin to take for granted the advantages you have achieved. You don't consider the fact that these advantages would vanish if you were to gain back weight. After Catherine had been following her new way of eating for a year, she forgot what it felt like to feel uncomfortable eating in public, how hard it had been to find well-fitting clothes, and how self-conscious she had been when she huffed and puffed climbing stairs. Like Catherine, once you begin to take such advantages for granted, you may repeatedly battle the sabotaging thought, *Is all this work really worth it?*

I want to assure you that most days and weeks and months and years will be relatively easy. But occasionally you will have a more difficult few days or weeks. At times you will experience more cravings, feel more deprived than usual, or tire of practicing your skills. Your life might become stressful, and when it does, it may not feel worth it to continue to put in the time and energy it takes to diet or maintain your weight loss.

This chapter will help you learn how to keep your motivation high throughout your life, regardless of what is going on around you. For the rest of your life, you will be following one of these three plans:

1. Daily Motivation Plan (page 188), when dieting or maintenance is going well

2. Re-Motivation Plan (page 191), when dieting or maintenance becomes difficult

3. Get-Back-on-Track Plan (page 198), when your skills slip and you gain weight

## Daily Motivation Plan

The Daily Motivation Plan will help you continually remind yourself that what you are doing to lose excess weight or to maintain your weight loss is so unquestionably worth it. You will do some of these skills every day for the rest of your life, and you will taper off doing others. The following shows you what to do throughout the day:

# each morning

Do the following each morning, before you eat breakfast:

**Prepare yourself as you get on the scale.** If you are maintaining at a weight that is higher than your dream weight, be careful what you say to yourself when you step on the scale. Imagine how you would feel and how burdensome maintenance eating would be if you always said to yourself, *I'm really disappointed ... I want to be thinner.* Then imagine how you would feel if you said, *This is great! I've lost _____ pounds since I started ... That's such an accomplishment ... Because of what I did and what I'm continuing to do, I'm healthier, I feel better about myself, I feel in control, I fit into clothes better, and I have more energy.* The former defeats you; the latter motivates you.

Make this following Response Card, post it by the scale, and prepare yourself each morning by reading it just before you weigh yourself:

> Remember the number I used to see when I got on the scale? The number I see now is great!

*Continue to read this card for a very long time and remind yourself of what it says for the rest of your life.*

**Fill in your graph.** If you are still losing weight, continue to notice how far you've come. If you are maintaining, give yourself credit when your weight is between the two red lines described on page 184. In a Cornell University study, maintainers who graphed their weight were more likely to hold steady, compared with participants in a control group.

*Continue to graph your weight for a very long time.*

**Review your Advantages Deck.** Keep reviewing your Advantages Deck daily until you are doing every skill in Stage 4, including following your plan without any struggle. But err on the side of caution: It's better to review your deck when you don't really need it than to skip reading it when you do. The moment you stop practicing a needed skill, deviate from your plan, or feel as if dieting has become more difficult, go back to reading your Advantages Deck daily. At some point, you can start reviewing the deck every other day, then once a week, then once every two weeks, and then once a month. You should stay at the once-a-month frequency for a very long time.

Now is also the time to modify your Advantages Deck. When you created it, you listed advantages that you hoped to achieve. Some of them may have come true for you already, and others may soon come true. As you read your deck, look for milestones you have already reached and rewrite those cards. For instance you might write, "I can walk two miles!" "I can buy clothes in regular stores!" "I don't have to take blood-pressure medication anymore!"

Also look for new advantages (although sometimes it's difficult to identify them because you have made gradual changes that you now may take for granted). For example, as we were problem-solving how Evelyn could find time to shop for groceries, I asked her, "I remember, when we first started working together, you told me you felt self-conscious at the supermarket because you thought people were looking in your cart and mentally criticizing you. Do you still feel like that?" Evelyn smiled and said, "No, never. I don't even think about it." I asked Evelyn to add that item to her Advantages Deck: "I feel fine at the grocery store, no matter what I put in my cart." Be on the lookout for experiences like this so you can add them to your deck.

*Continue to add to your Advantages Deck for a very long time.*

# several times a day

To do the following tasks, you may periodically need a visual reminder, such as putting on a bracelet you rarely wear, moving your watch to the other wrist, or wearing a rubber band around your wrist. Put a pop-up reminder on your computer or PDA, or make a note in your appointment book. When you notice the item or reminder, tell yourself what you need to do.

**Give yourself credit.** I find that many dieters gradually stop practicing this important skill as time goes on. You should be giving yourself credit throughout the entire day—at least 15 to 20 times, whenever you:

- Weigh yourself.

- Graph your weight.

- Read your Response Cards.

- Review your Advantages Deck.

- Eat slowly, while sitting down and enjoying every bite.

- Exercise.

- Think about your general eating plan for the day.

- Follow your plan for each meal and snack, or make appropriate modifications.

- Use Resistance Techniques.

- Tolerate hunger if it's not time to eat.

- Say no to tempting foods that are not on your plan.

- Contact your Diet Buddy.

You should also give yourself credit for giving yourself credit; filling out a Cheat Sheet as needed; being assertive with food pushers; making special requests at restaurants; postponing a meal or snack if you are upset; comforting yourself without food; making the time for diet and exercise activities; staying in control during special events; reading this book; adding to your Advantages Deck or making new Response Cards; writing cards for your Memory Box; and so on.

## *Continue giving yourself credit throughout your life.*

**Look for "worth-it" experiences.** You will have multiple opportunities every day to say to yourself, *It's so worth it to keep on going.* Every time you look in the mirror, say, *It's so worth it to look this way.* Every time you more easily accomplish a physical task—such as lugging heavy groceries—say, *It's so worth it.* Every time you realize a skill, such as ignoring a craving, has made your life easier, say, *This is really worth it.* When you recognize a repetitive worth-it experience, add it to your Advantages Deck.

*Continue to remind yourself why it's so worth it*
*for the rest of your life.*

# at the end of the day

Take a moment when you're feeling relaxed and calm to think about your day and then do the following:

**Add to your Memory Box.** Mentally review your day. Did you have any meaningful weight-loss or maintenance experiences? For example, Margaret wrote each of the following on a separate card:

- I walked up the long flight of stairs at the library without feeling winded.

- The nurse said my blood pressure is lower.

- My jeans are too big to wear.

- My neighbor says I'm shrinking.

*Continue to add to your Memory Box for the rest of your life.*


## Re-Motivation Plan

I've found that long-time dieters and maintainers go for a period of time (usually months) with little to no difficulty. Then, often without realizing it, they temporarily lose sight of what they have learned. They let some of their new eating behaviors slip. Then their weight goes up and their motivation goes down. They find themselves continually battling sabotaging thoughts, such as, *This is just too hard ... This isn't worth it ... I can't keep this up.* This happens to almost everyone from time to time. A dieter I counseled called it "maintainer's fatigue."

When dieting or maintaining feels harder, and especially whenever your "It's not worth it" thoughts become overly strong, it's time to temporarily step up your motivation efforts with this Re-Motivation Plan. Do the following daily—in addition to your Daily Motivation Plan—until dieting and maintaining feel worth it again.

**The first set of techniques will help you figure out the duration, frequency, and sources of your difficult times.**

**Add up the hard hours.** Be careful not to let a few difficult hours color the whole week. Ask yourself the following questions.

- *Does it seem too hard every hour of every day?*

- *When is it easier?*

- *How many hours was it really difficult?*

These questions will help you put things in perspective. Although it may feel as if you have been struggling all day long, chances are that there are still some hours and days when it's actually only mildly difficult, if at all. Recognizing that sticking to your plan is actually pretty easy most of the time motivates you to persevere during the more difficult minutes or hours.

**Analyze why you are having a harder time.** Perhaps it is due to circumstances that can be changed. For example, maybe you are working longer hours and need to delegate more tasks to your family. Maybe you haven't made getting to the store and preparing your food a priority. Ask yourself:

- *In which situations is it harder?*

- *Do I need to do some problem solving?*

Difficulties may have arisen due to your eating behavior. Ask yourself:

- *Am I still eating as nutritiously as before?*

- *Am I still eating everything slowly, while sitting down and enjoying every bite?*

- *Should I time my snacks differently?*

- *Should I vary the foods I eat (still using the Think Thin Formula)?*

- *Have I stopped saying to myself, NO CHOICE? Am I struggling over which food to eat?*

**Consider whether you are eating too little.** Dieting becomes harder than it needs to be if you are trying to sustain a calorie level that is too low for your appetite and life circumstances. It's fine to make the decision to go up to the next calorie level if you are struggling. You may gain a couple of pounds, but it may be a relief to be able to eat a little more. If you think this may be the case, it's probably worth at least trying the next calorie level. If you find it doesn't make a difference or you're too unhappy with the weight gain, you can always go back to your previous calorie level and the extra weight will come off.

**Check on your level of acceptance.** Some dieters or maintainers get to the point where they ask, "You mean, I have to eat this way for the rest of my life!?" They may have understood intellectually from the beginning that they had to change their eating for good, but they didn't really grasp it on an emotional level, so they struggle.

Remind yourself often that you can eat what you want, whenever you want, in any quantities you want—or you can be thinner. But you can't have it both ways. Also remember that it was easier before and it will get easier again. And when it is easier, there's probably no question in your mind that it's worth it.

**Monitor your level of general self-care.** Make sure your life is in balance: Are you engaging in enough pleasurable activities? It's important to get satisfaction from non-food sources. Do you need to reduce your stress? Are you getting enough sleep? Everything is harder if you don't get enough non-food satisfaction, you're stressed, or you're tired.

**The next few techniques will remind you what will happen if you abandon your efforts.**

**Remember the old you.** Remind yourself what life was like when you were heavier and unhappy about it. What was a typical day like for you? How did you feel physically? Visualize a specific experience or event that encapsulates the negative consequences of being heavier. For example, maybe your weight overshadowed what could have been a pleasant experience at a party or at the beach. Picture it in your mind: What were you wearing? Whom were you with? How did you feel about your appearance? What did you think others were thinking about you? Were you worried about what you were going to eat, how you would stay in control, and how others would view your food choices? Ask yourself, *Do I really want to go back to that?*

**Recall the old feelings.** Think about the last time you gained back weight. Did you feel guilty about eating foods you knew you shouldn't have? Were you unhappy, frustrated, and angry with yourself? Did you feel out of control and hopeless? Unfortunately, this is undoubtedly how you will feel again if you stop following your plan and regain the weight you lost. Avoiding this kind of distress (which could become permanent) is a good reason to keep going.

**Visualize the future if you gain weight.** Imagine, in great detail, the most likely scenario if you go back to your old way of eating: Can you see yourself getting heavier? Can you imagine how you will feel when you see the number on the scale going up ... and up ... and up? Can you picture having to put away your smaller clothes and getting out your bigger ones—the clothes you had promised yourself you would never have to wear again?

Now visualize the future if you keep following the Beck Diet for Life Program. Imagine a specific event you have coming up (perhaps a wedding, vacation, party, or business meeting) and think about how great you will feel if you have kept your weight down. Picture it in your mind: What will you wear? Whom will you talk to? How much more comfortable will you feel at your new weight?

**The following techniques will help you respond to your sabotaging thoughts.**

**Remind yourself that the difficult times are temporary.** Dieting or maintaining, like many things in life, is sometimes easier and sometimes harder. It's supposed to be that way. Don't get too worried. As long as you keep pushing through, this difficult time will definitely pass. There are many techniques in this chapter that you can use to make it pass even sooner.

**Respond strongly to your "It's not worth it" thoughts.** When this idea is strong in your mind and your resolve is weak, remind yourself that this is a *toxic* thought. You will be so glad later that you didn't give in to it! Recall other experiences when you had that thought but persevered anyway. For example, have you ever thought, *It's not worth it,* when you had to study for an important exam or when you were holding yourself to a budget to save money for a vacation? Did it turn out to be worth it? Dieting may seem hard right now, but remember when it was so much easier? It will get easier again.

Make a Response Card:

> It's hard now, but hard times are normal and always pass. As long as I keep going, it will get easier again. It's worth it!

**Respond to your disappointment.** Some dieters become disappointed when they realize that their maintenance weight is higher than they hoped it would be. They become less motivated, questioning whether they should have even dieted in the first place. This is an example of all-or-nothing thinking: *Either I get to the weight I wanted (regardless of the fact that it was unrealistic in the first place) or I shouldn't* *have put in the effort to try at all.* If this happens to you, ask yourself, *Do I view other goals in this way?* If you can't become the best tennis player or guitarist or runner, does it mean you shouldn't have taken it up in the first place? Of course not! Now, more than ever, you need to see what advantages you have achieved, or at least partially achieved. Even if you can't fit into the size you had hoped for, would you rather be limited to the clothes you were wearing before you started the Beck Diet for Life Program? Even if you haven't achieved every physiological benefit, would you trade your current state of health for what it used to be?

**Make a Response Card about dealing with stress.** If old sabotaging thoughts about deserving or needing to eat when you are under stress resurface, make the following card:

> Stress is a normal part of life. It comes and goes. If I go back to coping with stress by eating, I will feel even worse. My stress will eventually diminish. When it does, do I want to be heavier?

**Beware of fears.** Some dieters get worried as they lose more and more weight. They sometimes have sabotaging thoughts such as, *What if people start to pay more attention to me or are attracted to me? ... If I get thinner, I won't have an excuse to avoid [a challenge, such as dating, being assertive with others, getting physically active] ... If I get to such-and-such weight, I won't know who I am ... What if people start to have greater expectations of me and I can't live up to them?* These dire predictions can interfere with your motivation to continue. If you have thoughts like these, recognize that you're thinking of the *worst* outcome (and you're not considering other scenarios). Ask yourself the following questions:

- *That's the worst-case scenario. If it happened, how would I cope?*

- *What's the best that could happen in this scenario?*

- *What's the most realistic outcome of this scenario?*

Answering these questions should help reduce your anxiety. Mandy, for example, was concerned that if she got thinner, she would get more male attention. We talked about specific situations she was afraid might arise (a man at a bar trying to persuade her to have another drink or leave with him; a blind date that wasn't turning out well). We role-played what she could say in these situations, and her fears decreased significantly when she realized that she could handle them.

Ben was afraid that he wouldn't know who he was if he lost weight because he had been overweight his whole life. We discussed how the core of who he was wouldn't be different, just the package it was presented in. I asked him if it was worth it to work on accepting this new version of himself if it meant he got to be happier, healthier, and thinner in return. He answered yes, it definitely was.

**The following techniques will help you remember why it's so worth it to keep up your efforts.**

**Add more cards to your Advantages Deck.** Ask yourself the following questions and see if they can help you come up with more cards to put in your deck. As a result of being thinner:

- *What can I do now that I couldn't do before?*

- *What can I do more easily?*

- *What am I less reluctant to do?*

- *Which activities/experiences do I get greater satisfaction from?*

- *When do I feel less self-conscious?*

- *When do I feel less guilty?*

- *When do I feel less anxious?*

- *When do I feel less embarrassed?*

- *When do I feel better about myself?*

- *In which situations do I feel more confident?*

- *How has my health changed?*

- *How has my body changed?*

- *How has my mindset changed?*

**Pull out your "big" jeans.** Keep an old pair of pants or a sweater in the front of your closet, one that you wore before you started the Beck Diet for Life Program.

Every morning when you get dressed, remind yourself of how absolutely terrific it is that you now wear a new size. Give yourself the same reminder every time you go shopping for clothes.

**Click off "worth-it" experiences.** Instead of just noting these experiences, use a counter (the one I suggested you use on page 67 to count off how often you deserve credit). For at least a week, click the counter every time you experience a weight-loss benefit.

For example, Toni clicked her counter when she:

- Stepped on the scale and thought about the number she used to see—Click!
- Looked in the mirror in the morning—Click!
- Got dressed in smaller-sized clothing—Click!
- Climbed the basement steps more easily—Click!
- Got out of the car more easily—Click!
- Felt confident at a meeting—Click!
- Lifted heavier weights at the gym—Click!
- Pedaled the stationary bike for half an hour—Click!
- Bought regular-sized panty hose—Click!
- Passed a bakery and didn't even think about going inside—Click!
- Easily walked fast to get to a movie on time—Click!
- Felt good about passing up popcorn at the movies—Click!

In addition to these experiences, Toni also clicked her counter multiple times a day when she felt good about the food she had eaten and when she felt in control: click, click, click, click, click, click!

Every time you click your counter, say to yourself, *This makes it worth it,* which is shorthand for, *I'm so glad to have this experience ... I want to continue having experiences like this ... I'm going to keep doing what I need to do so I can continue.*

**Look at your entire weight-loss progress.** Tape your graphs together so you can see how far you've come since the beginning.

**Call your Diet Buddy.** Ask for help with problem solving and motivation. Talk with your buddy about what feels difficult and get his/her advice. Go through the Re-Motivation techniques with your buddy, who can reinforce the merits of continuing to diet or maintain, and can help you think of more ways that it is all worth it.

# Get-Back-on-Track Plan

## in session with Dr. Beck

Jamie, who had originally lost 37 pounds, came back to see me three years after our last session. She had gained back 8 pounds over three months, starting around Thanksgiving. Jamie had tried to get back on track, but she couldn't seem to start losing weight again.

**Jamie:** I don't know what's wrong. I've been trying.

**Dr. Beck:** Well, let's go down the list: Have you been looking at your Advantages Deck every day? Reading your Response Cards? Eating everything slowly, while sitting down and enjoying every bite? Giving yourself credit?

**Jamie:** Not really, not every day.

**Dr. Beck:** Well, no wonder you're having trouble. Are some sabotaging thoughts getting in your way?

**Jamie:** It just seems like it will take so much effort.

**Dr. Beck:** Well, it *will* take a lot of effort—at first. Tell me, do you remember when you first came to see me? Was it hard at first, when you were learning new skills?

**Jamie:** Yes, I remember some things were pretty hard in the beginning.

**Dr. Beck:** And did they stay hard?

**Jamie:** No, everything got much easier. In fact, it's been pretty easy this whole time. I mean, I've had days here and there that were hard. Like when I got sick last summer, it was hard. But I was always able to get right back on track. I don't know what happened this time.

**Dr. Beck:** Well, from what you've said, it sounds as if you got derailed by the holidays. Then you started practicing some of the skills you had let slip, but a sabotaging thought got in the way: *This is taking too much effort.* I think you weren't able to talk back to that thought, and so it made it so much harder to try to use your skills. Do you think that's what happened?

**Jamie:** That sounds about right.

**Dr. Beck:** And how about this thought: *It will take too much effort.* Do you think that's completely true?

**Jamie:** No, I guess not. It probably will get easier. And I really don't want to go back to the way it was before I lost weight.

**Dr. Beck:** Should we work on getting you to motivate yourself to do the work?

**Jamie:** Yes, I definitely want to lose this extra weight. I really don't feel very good.

**Dr. Beck:** Okay, then, let's start. Can we go over your advantages of losing weight again?

Once Jamie got back to practicing her Stages 1 and 2 skills (including planning all of her meals for a week and sticking to her plans inflexibly), the number on the scale started to go down, her confidence went up, and her motivation increased dramatically until she lost all of the weight she had regained.

Some long-time dieters and maintainers occasionally get way off track, not just for an evening, but for several weeks. Their *I don't care* or *I can't do it anymore* sabotaging thoughts get overpoweringly strong. They gain back some weight, and all of the old negative feelings kick back in. They feel discouraged, disappointed, angry, pessimistic, and helpless.

But regaining some weight is to be expected. Relapse is normal. Mistakes are normal. Falling off the wagon isn't the end of the world. And it can be much easier than you might imagine to climb back on. Charlie told me the following analogy, which I thought was wonderful: When you fall off the wagon, it doesn't take off without you; it sits there, next to you, waiting for you to climb back on. As long as you go back to using your skills, you don't lose everything you've worked so hard to achieve. And you have a lot to gain if you can learn how to analyze and learn from your mistakes.

Do the following to get back on track:

**Avoid turning a relapse into a catastrophe.** You will make a relapse worse if you tell yourself, *This is terrible ... I can't believe I let this happen ... I'm so weak ... I can't get back in control ... What's the use of even trying? I'm going to gain back all of the weight I lost, like I did all of the other times.* You will make the situation better if you tell yourself, *Okay, so I gained back some weight ... As long as I recommit now, it's just not a big deal ... In retrospect, this was predictable ... I stopped using some of my skills ... But they worked before, and they'll work now ... Besides, learning them for the first time was the really hard part ... Now that I already know them, getting back to them will be easier.* Then commit to doing everything possible to regain control.

**Give yourself credit.** Are you thinking, *I went off track ... What could I deserve credit for?* You deserve a lot of credit for catching yourself. You could have let it go even longer and gained even more weight.

**Recall your past experiences.** Think about a specific time when you were actively losing weight. Remind yourself:

- How good you felt when you were using the Success Skills every day

- How easy dieting became

- How proud you were of yourself

Then reflect on how much easier it will be the second time around because you already know that the Beck Diet for Life Program works and you already know that you can do it.

**Go back to Phase 1.** Remind yourself how easy it had become to practice these skills. Return to implementing them daily:

1. Go back to making a written plan the night before and sticking to it exactly. You may need to do this just for a few days or for a few weeks before you return to flexible eating. Build your confidence that you can return to being 100 percent in control of your eating.

2. Make sure you eat *everything* slowly, while sitting down and enjoying every bite. If you have been making any exceptions to these skills, don't give yourself a choice about them now.

3. Think ahead of time about the foods you will need to stick to your plan, how you're going to get them, and when you're going to prepare them.

4. Make an effort to eat more meals at home for a couple of days or weeks so that you know exactly what you're eating and are not taking in any "hidden" calories.

5. If you have stopped weighing yourself, get back on the scale every morning! Graph your weight again until it comes back down.

6. If you have been lax about exercising, make sure you recommit to a firm exercise plan and don't give yourself a choice about sticking to it.

7. Give yourself credit for every positive diet- and exercise-related behavior.

8. Go back to checking in with your Diet Buddy daily.

Finally, fill out a Stage 5 Success Skills Sheet (pages 274–275) every night without fail. You will feel so much more in control.

**Respond to your sabotaging thoughts.** If you are reluctant to return to Stage 1 and get started again, it is probably because you are having the following thoughts:

- *It's too much trouble.*

- *I can get back on track without doing the skills.*

- *I already know what I need to do.*

You will need to firmly remind yourself of how helpful the Beck Diet for Life Program was the first time around. If you don't go back to Stage 1 and refresh your skills, you will put yourself at high risk for continuing to struggle and gain weight.

Don't give yourself a choice about it. Taking the first step — starting to reread Chapter 4—will probably be the hardest. Once you begin, you will like the feeling of regaining control, and it will be so much easier to keep going.

**Learn from your mistakes.** Think about how you got off track: What do you wish you had done differently? What do you want to do next time? Write a letter to your future self in your Diet Notebook under the heading "Get-Back-on-Track Letter." Read Gail's letter to her future self and use it as a guide for creating your own:

Get-Back-on-Track Letter

Okay, you got off track again. No big deal. You gained back some weight. But don't get scared. Don't get hopeless. You were probably stressed, traveling, or celebrating. It's good that you're reading this letter now, before you regain even more weight. You know what to do. You did it before, and you can do it now.

Remember how good you felt on your last birthday? It was great. Compared with your birthday the year before, you were much thinner. You were proud of yourself! Bill and Alyssa were so surprised when they saw you. You stayed on the dance floor all night. You didn't feel heavy and self-conscious. You loved the outfit you wore. You didn't mind not drinking. You were happy to have just a small piece of cake. You didn't feel deprived. You felt in control. You felt GREAT.

You can get to that place again. It won't be as hard as the first time. Go read the book and start checking off the Success Skills Sheet every day. Start right now. You will be SO happy you did!

It is important for you to know that maintaining your weight loss will likely be cyclical. You get down to your maintenance weight, and then you may gradually loosen up some, without even recognizing what you are doing. You gain a little, go back to consciously using your skills, and then lose the extra weight again. The number on the scale will continue to tell you exactly how you're doing. Over time, you will learn from these small peaks and valleys. You will get back on track sooner. You will use your skills more and more effectively, and you will develop the confidence to know you *can* get back in control. And you will have lots of experiences that prove how much better you feel when you do.

# chapter 9

# Where to Go from Here

You've come to the end of *The Complete Beck Diet for Life,* but you should use this book as a resource over and over again to help keep yourself on track. Using your skills and choosing healthful foods will continue to get easier over time. Realistically, though, you will always have to remain vigilant. You will periodically have to tolerate at least a little hunger, as everyone without a weight problem does.

Desire and cravings will never completely go away, either. As a long-time successful maintainer, I still experience them. For example, one evening as I was working on this manuscript, I had the thought, *I'm hungry ... Maybe I'll go down to the kitchen and get something to eat.* But I didn't, because I talked back to myself: *Now, wait a minute ... You just finished dinner an hour and a half ago ... It's not time to eat, and your stomach doesn't even feel empty ... You just want to eat because you don't feel like working ... You're having some trouble concentrating because you haven't taken a break for a while ... Don't go into the kitchen ... E-mail a friend instead.* So I did, and I was immediately glad that I hadn't strayed from my plan. After a few minutes, the desire to eat went away completely.

Continue to practice all of your Success Skills consistently, long after you reach the maintenance stage. You will need to use some skills for the rest of your life. No matter how motivated you feel and no matter how easy weight maintenance may seem, *always* weigh yourself daily; faithfully do planned exercise and take advantage of spontaneous exercise; use your Resistance Techniques; practice good eating habits at every meal and snack (eating everything slowly, while sitting down and enjoying every bite); continually give yourself credit for all of the things you do right; and recommit *right away* whenever you make a mistake.

Over time, you will probably find that you automatically start using some of these skills in other areas of your life. For example, many dieters have told me that for the first time they found that they were also able to overcome such challenges as smoking, overspending, and procrastinating. They were able to manage their time better and to organize their households and work lives. They learned how to set goals and steadily work toward them.

How did this happen?

- They learned how to exert self-control. They learned how to do what they needed to do, instead of what they *felt* like doing at the moment.

- They learned how to anticipate problems and to solve them in advance.

- They learned how to be accountable to themselves.

- They learned how to tolerate negative emotions.

- They learned how to give themselves credit and build their confidence.

- They learned how to talk back to their sabotaging thoughts.

- They learned how to persist in the face of difficulty.

- They learned what to do when they felt a sense of unfairness.

- They learned how to recover from mistakes.

- They learned how to feel entitled to take care of themselves and to be assertive with others.

- They learned how to ask for help when they needed it.

It is my hope that you will always be mindful of the wonderful benefits you have gained from losing weight and that you will always be appreciative of all of the other positive aspects of your day-to-day experiences. Continue to enrich your life. Try making a list of goals that you would like to accomplish: Do you want to volunteer your time, improve your career, meet new people, pursue new interests, or travel more? Do you want to enhance your spirituality, creativity, knowledge, or relationships? Make a plan to start working toward these goals. What should your first step be? Take the skills you have learned from *The Complete Beck Diet for Life* and use them to improve your whole life.

*************

Finally, as I mentioned in the Introduction, I learn so much from dieters who e-mail me about their experiences. Please visit www.beckdietforlife.com to contact me or find additional resources to help you with your weight-loss and maintenance journey.

# Part 3

# chapter 10

# Think Thin Formulas & Food Lists

I n this chapter, you'll find everything you need to follow the Think Thin Initial and Lifetime Eating Plans. First, determine which calorie level is right for you (page 107). Next, find the corresponding Think Thin Formula (pages 210–214). Then look through the 11 Think Thin Food Lists:

- **Breakfast Options** (page 215)
- **Lunch Options** (pages 216–217)
- **Dinner Options** (page 218)
- **Starter Salad and Soup Options** (page 219)
- **Fruit Options** (page 220)
- **Vegetable Options** (page 221)
- **Grain and Starch Side Dish Options** (pages 222–223)
- **Snack Options** (page 224)
- **Condiment and Accompaniment Options** (page 225)
- **Add-On Options** (page 225)
- **Bonus Calorie Options** (pages 226–227)

The recipes in Chapter 11 provide you with additional selections.

> **On the Think Thin Eating Plan, you can eat an appropriate amount of any food you desire. Nothing is off-limits.** If a category doesn't include a food you like (or a particular version), check the nutrition label or use a calorie counter to figure out the appropriate portion size and add it to the list.

Please note these guidelines. They are so important that I have put a box before each one for you to check after you have read it.

☐ Check nutrition labels to make sure you are eating the correct portion for your allotted calories. Brands vary, and manufacturers change their products.

☐ Measure carefully. Extra calories will slow your weight loss.

☐ For more flexibility and variety, choose any two ½ servings of food (instead of a full portion) from the same list (except for multicomponent options). For example, instead of a full serving of yogurt at breakfast, you could have a ½ serving of yogurt and a ½ serving of cheese. In some cases, I have indicated for you to do this yourself. You'll see a smaller portion of food and then "plus ½ item from this list."

☐ Many recipes from Chapter 11 (pages 228–262) are complete or semi-complete meals, and as a result, are not paired with side dishes or Add-On Calories. Check your Think Thin Formula.

☐ Some foods, such as milk or squash, can be found in more than one list of food.

☐ Try a wide variety of foods, especially new ones, to discover which ones you find most enjoyable and filling.

☐ If you'd like to add extra ingredients or an extra portion of food, use Bonus Calories.

☐ Have the equivalent of at least 2 cups each of fruit and dairy products a day.

☐ Dairy products are often available in non-fat, low-fat, and full-fat versions. Check product labels if you would like a version not included in the food lists.

☐ Limit your intake of saturated fats but include healthy fats, which can keep you feeling satiated for longer (e.g., omega-3 fatty acids found in flaxseed and some fish and vegetables, or monounsaturated fats found in olives, nuts, and avocado).

☐ Check with your health-care professional about other foods you may need to limit (e.g., eggs, red meat, items high in salt, fish with mercury, and soy). Also check to see if you should be taking additional calcium or vitamins.

☐ All applicable protein items are cooked, skinless and boneless, and have been trimmed of visible fat.

# 2,400-*Calorie Think Thin Formula*

**Breakfast:** 350 calories   **Lunch:** 650 calories   **Dinner:** 750 calories
**Snacks:** 3 (150-calorie) snacks   **Bonus Calories:** 200 calories

## Breakfast Options: 350 calories total

**Main Dish:**

**1** (250-calorie) Breakfast Option
(page 215)

**Side Dish:**

**1** (100-calorie) fruit
**or**
**1** (100-calorie) grain/starch

································ **OR** ································

**1** (250-calorie) Breakfast Recipe
(pages 230–232)

**1** (100-calorie) fruit
**or**
**1** (100-calorie) grain/starch

## Lunch Options: 650 calories total

**Main Dish:**

**1** (250-calorie)
Lunch Option
(page 217)

**Side Dish:**

**1** (100-calorie) fruit
**and**
**1** (150-calorie) grain/starch

**Plus:**

**1** (50-calorie) soup **or** salad **or** vegetable
**and**
**1** (50-calorie) Add-On Option
**and**
**1** (50-calorie) vegetable

································ **OR** ································

**Main Dish:**

**1** (350-calorie)
Lunch Recipe
(pages 234–236
and 256–258)

**Side Dish:**

**1** (100-calorie) fruit
**and**
**1** (100-calorie) grain/starch

**Plus:**

**1** (50-calorie) soup **or** salad **or** vegetable
**and**
**1** (50-calorie) vegetable

## Dinner Options: 750 calories total

**Main Dish:**

**1** (300-calorie)
Dinner Option
(page 218)

**Side Dish:**

**1** (100-calorie) fruit
**and**
**1** (150-calorie) grain/starch

**Plus:**

**1** (50-calorie) soup **or** salad **or** vegetable
**and**
**1** (50-calorie) Add-On Option
**and**
**2** (50-calorie) vegetables

································ **OR** ································

**Main Dish:**

**1** (450-calorie)
Dinner Recipe
(pages 237–247
and 259–262)

**Side Dish:**

**1** (100-calorie) fruit
**and**
**1** (100-calorie) grain/starch

**Plus:**

**1** (50-calorie) soup **or** salad **or** vegetable
**and**
**1** (50-calorie) vegetable

# 2,200-*Calorie Think Thin Formula*

**Breakfast:** 350 calories   **Lunch:** 500 calories   **Dinner:** 700 calories
**Snacks:** 3 (150-calorie) snacks   **Bonus Calories:** 200 calories

## Breakfast Options: 350 calories total

**Main Dish:**

**1** (250-calorie) Breakfast Option
(page 215)

**Side Dish:**

**1** (100-calorie) fruit
**or**
**1** (100-calorie) grain/starch

···············································OR············································

**1** (250-calorie) Breakfast Recipe
(pages 230–232)

**1** (100-calorie) fruit
**or**
**1** (100-calorie) grain/starch

## Lunch Options: 500 calories total

**Main Dish:**

**1** (250-calorie)
Lunch Option
(page 217)

**Side Dish:**

**1** (100-calorie) fruit
**or**
**1** (100-calorie) grain/starch

**Plus:**

**1** (50-calorie) soup **or** salad **or**
vegetable
**and**
**1** (50-calorie) Add-On Option
**and**
**1** (50-calorie) vegetable

···············································OR············································

**Main Dish:**

**1** (300-calorie)
Lunch Recipe
(pages 234–236
and 256–258)

**Side Dish:**

**1** (100-calorie) fruit
**or**
**1** (100-calorie) grain/starch

**Plus:**

**1** (50-calorie) soup **or** salad **or**
vegetable
**and**
**1** (50-calorie) vegetable

## Dinner Options: 700 calories total

**Main Dish:**

**1** (300-calorie)
Dinner Option
(page 218)

**Side Dish:**

**1** (100-calorie) fruit
**and**
**1** (150-calorie) grain/starch

**Plus:**

**1** (50-calorie) soup **or** salad **or**
vegetable
**and**
**1** (50-calorie) Add-On Option
**and**
**1** (50-calorie) vegetable

···············································OR············································

**Main Dish:**

**1** (450-calorie)
Dinner Recipe
(pages 237–247
and 259–262)

**Side Dish:**

**1** (100-calorie) fruit
**or**
**1** (100-calorie) grain/starch

**Plus:**

**1** (50-calorie) soup **or** salad **or**
vegetable
**and**
**1** (50-calorie) Add-On Option
**and**
**1** (50-calorie) vegetable

# 2,000-*Calorie Think Thin Formula*

**Breakfast:** 350 calories  **Lunch:** 500 calories  **Dinner:** 550 calories
**Snacks:** 3 (150-calorie) snacks  **Bonus Calories:** 150 calories

## Breakfast Options: 350 calories total

**Main Dish:**

**1** (250-calorie) Breakfast Option
(page 215)

**Side Dish:**

**1** (100-calorie) fruit
**or**
**1** (100-calorie) grain/starch

·····**OR**·····

**1** (250-calorie) Breakfast Recipe
(pages 230–232)

**1** (100-calorie) fruit
**or**
**1** (100-calorie) grain/starch

## Lunch Options: 500 calories total

**Main Dish:**

**1** (250-calorie)
Lunch Option
(page 217)

**Side Dish:**

**1** (100-calorie) fruit
**or**
**1** (100-calorie) grain/starch

**Plus:**

**1** (50-calorie) soup **or** salad **or**
vegetable
**and**
**1** (50-calorie) Add-On Option
**and**
**1** (50-calorie) vegetable

·····**OR**·····

**Main Dish:**

**1** (300-calorie)
Lunch Recipe
(pages 234–236
and 256–258)

**Side Dish:**

**1** (100-calorie) fruit
**or**
**1** (100-calorie) grain/starch

**Plus:**

**1** (50-calorie) soup **or** salad **or**
vegetable
**and**
**1** (50-calorie) vegetable

## Dinner Options: 550 calories total

**Main Dish:**

**1** (300-calorie)
Dinner Option
(page 218)

**Side Dish:**

**1** (100-calorie) fruit
**or**
**1** (100-calorie) grain/starch

**Plus:**

**1** (50-calorie) soup **or** salad **or**
vegetable
**and**
**1** (50-calorie) Add-On Option
**and**
**1** (50-calorie) vegetable

·····**OR**·····

**Main Dish:**

**1** (450-calorie)
Dinner Recipe
(pages 237–247
and 259–262)

**Side Dish:**

**1** (50-calorie) soup **or** salad **or**
vegetable

**Plus:**

**1** (50-calorie) vegetable

# 1,800-*Calorie Think Thin Formula*

**Breakfast:** 350 calories   **Lunch:** 450 calories   **Dinner:** 550 calories
**Snacks:** 3 (100-calorie) snacks   **Bonus Calories:** 150 calories

## Breakfast Options: 350 calories total

**Main Dish:**

**1** (250-calorie) Breakfast Option
(page 215)

**Side Dish:**

**1** (100-calorie) fruit
**or**
**1** (100-calorie) grain/starch

·······OR·······

**1** (250-calorie) Breakfast Recipe
(pages 230–232)

**1** (100-calorie) fruit
**or**
**1** (100-calorie) grain/starch

## Lunch Options: 450 calories total

**Main Dish:**

**1** (250-calorie)
Lunch Option
(page 217)

**Side Dish:**

**1** (100-calorie) fruit
**or**
**1** (100-calorie) grain/starch

**Plus:**

**1** (50-calorie) soup **or** salad **or**
vegetable
**and**
**1** (50-calorie) vegetable
**or**
**1** (50-calorie) Add-On Option

·······OR·······

**Main Dish:**

**1** (350-calorie)
Lunch Recipe
(pages 234–236
and 256–258)

**Side Dish:**

**1** (50-calorie) soup **or** salad **or**
vegetable

**Plus:**

**1** (50-calorie) vegetable
**or**
**1** (50-calorie) Add-On Option

## Dinner Options: 550 calories total

**Main Dish:**

**1** (300-calorie)
Dinner Option
(page 217)

**Side Dish:**

**1** (100-calorie) fruit
**or**
**1** (100-calorie) grain/starch

**Plus:**

**1** (50-calorie) soup **or** salad **or**
vegetable
**and**
**1** (50-calorie) Add-On Option
**and**
**1** (50-calorie) vegetable

·······OR·······

**Main Dish:**

**1** (450-calorie)
Dinner Recipe
(pages 237–247
and 259–262)

**Side Dish:**

**1** (50-calorie) soup **or** salad **or**
vegetable

**Plus:**

**1** (50-calorie) vegetable

# 1,600-*Calorie Think Thin Formula*

**Breakfast:** 250 calories  **Lunch:** 400 calories  **Dinner:** 500 calories

**Snacks:** 3 (100-calorie) snacks  **Bonus Calories:** 150 calories

## Breakfast Options: 250 calories total

**Main Dish:**

**1** (150-calorie) Breakfast Option
 (page 215)

**Side Dish:**

**1** (100-calorie) fruit
or
**1** (100-calorie) grain/starch

········································OR········································

**1** (250-calorie) Breakfast Recipe
(pages 230–232)

## Lunch Options: 400 calories total

**Main Dish:**

**1** (200-calorie)
Lunch Option
(page 216)

**Side Dish:**

**1** (100-calorie) fruit
or
**1** (100-calorie) grain/starch

**Plus:**

**1** (50-calorie) soup or salad or
vegetable
and
**1** (50-calorie) vegetable
or
**1** (50-calorie) Add-On Option

········································OR········································

**Main Dish:**

**1** (300-calorie)
Lunch Recipe
(pages 234–236
and 256–258)

**Side Dish:**

**1** (50-calorie) soup or salad or
vegetable

**Plus:**

**1** (50-calorie) vegetable
or
**1** (50-calorie) Add-On Option

## Dinner Options: 500 calories total

**Main Dish:**

**1** (300-calorie)
Dinner Option
(page 218)

**Side Dish:**

**1** (100-calorie) fruit
or
**1** (100-calorie) grain/starch

**Plus:**

**1** (50-calorie) soup or salad or
vegetable
and
**1** (50-calorie) vegetable
or
**1** (50-calorie) Add-On Option

········································OR········································

**Main Dish:**

**1** (400-calorie)
Dinner Recipe
(pages 237–247
and 259–262)

**Side Dish:**

**1** (50-calorie) soup or salad or
vegetable

**Plus:**

**1** (50-calorie) vegetable

# Think Thin Food Lists
## Breakfast Options (Protein)

| 150-Calorie Portions | 250-Calorie Portions |
|---|---|
| • Bacon, turkey, 4 oz | • Bacon, turkey, 3.3 oz **plus** ½ item from this list |
| • Breakfast cereal, with at least 8g protein and 6g fiber (check label for 100-calorie portion size) **plus** ½ cup skim or soy milk | • Breakfast cereal, with at least 8g protein and 6g fiber (check label for 150-calorie portion size) **plus** 1 cup skim or soy milk |
| • Cheese, cottage, 1% (1 cup) or 4% (⅔ cup) | • Cheese, cottage, 1% (1⅔ cups) or 4% (1 cup) |
| • Cheese, farmer's, 2 oz | • Cheese, farmer's, 3.3 oz |
| • Cheese, goat, 1.5 oz | • Cheese, goat, 2.5 oz |
| • Cheese, hard, 1.2 oz | • Cheese, hard, 2 oz |
| • Cheese, ricotta, fat-free (1 cup) or part-skim (½ cup) | • Cheese, ricotta, fat-free (1⅔ cups) or part-skim (¾ cup) |
| • Chicken or turkey, cooked, 3 oz | • Chicken or turkey, cooked, 5 oz |
| • Cream cheese, regular (1½ Tbsp) **plus** ½ item from this list | • Cream cheese, regular, 2½ Tbsp **plus** ½ item from this list |
| • Cream cheese, whipped or low-fat (2 Tbsp) **plus** ½ item from this list | • Cream cheese, whipped or low-fat, 3⅓ Tbsp |
| • Eggs, 2 | • Eggs, 3 |
| • Egg whites, 4 **plus** ½ item from this list | • Egg whites, 6½ **plus** ½ item from this list |
| • Egg substitute, ½ cup **plus** ½ item from this list | • Egg substitute, ¾ cup **plus** ½ item from this list |
| • Milk, skim, ¾ cup **plus** ½ item from this list | • Nut butters; peanut, almond, or cashew; 2½ Tbsp |
| • Nut butters; peanut, almond, or cashew; 1½ Tbsp | • Oatmeal, cooked with water, 1 cup **plus** 1 cup skim or soy milk |
| • Oatmeal, cooked with water, 1 cup | • Sausage, chicken, 5 oz **or** turkey, 3.7 oz |
| • Sausage, chicken, 3 oz **or** turkey, 2.2 oz | • Smoked salmon, 3.7 oz **plus** ½ item from this list |
| • Smoked salmon, 4.5 oz | • Yogurt, plain, non-fat (1¾ cups) or low-fat (1⅔ cups) |
| • Yogurt, plain, non-fat (1⅛ cups) or low-fat (1 cup) | • Yogurt, flavored or full-fat (check label) |
| • Yogurt, flavored or full-fat (check label) | |

# Think Thin Food Lists
## Lunch Options (Protein)

## 200-Calorie Portions

### Meat and Poultry:

- Beef brisket or corned beef brisket, 2.8 oz
- Beef, ground or hamburger, 90% lean, 3 oz
- Chicken, breast, 4 oz
- Chicken burger or sausage, or ground chicken, 3.5 oz
- Deli: chicken breast, ham, turkey breast, or roast beef, 5 oz
- Ham, sirloin steak, or veal loin, 4 oz
- Hotdog, beef, 2 oz
- Hotdog, beef, 97% fat-free, 4 oz **plus** ½ item from this list
- Turkey, breast, 3.8 oz
- Turkey burger or hotdog or sausage, or ground turkey, 3 oz

### Dairy:

- Cheese, cottage, 1% (1⅓ cups) or 4% (⅞ cup)
- Cheese, farmer's, 2.5 oz
- Cheese, goat, 2 oz
- Cheese, hard, 1.8 oz
- Cheese, ricotta, fat-free (1⅓ cups) or part-skim (⅔ cup)
- Eggs, 2½
- Egg whites, 5 **plus** ½ item from this list
- Milk, skim, 1 cup **plus** ½ item from this list
- Yogurt, plain, non-fat (1½ cups) or low-fat (1⅓ cups)
- Yogurt, flavored or full-fat (check label)

### Fish and Seafood:

- Calamari, crab, lobster, oysters, shrimp, or scallops, 6.6 oz
- Cod, flounder, tilapia, or sole, 6 oz
- Imitation crab, 6.5 oz
- Salmon, cooked, 4 oz or canned, 5 oz
- Smoked salmon, 3 oz **plus** ½ item from this list
- Sushi (pick 2 of these 3 choices):
  - 2.5 pieces eel roll or California roll
  - 3 pieces tuna roll or salmon roll
  - 4.5 pieces cucumber roll
- Swordfish, 5 oz
- Tuna, cooked, 4 oz or chunk light canned, 7 oz

### Vegetarian:

- Beans or lentils, cooked, 6 oz
- Chili, canned (check label)
- Hummus, ½ cup
- Nut butters; peanut, almond, or cashew; 2 Tbsp
- Pizza, 2.3 oz (1 slice of 14-inch thin-crust, plain)
- Seitan, 4.6 oz
- Tahini, 2 Tbsp
- Tempeh, uncooked, 3.5 oz
- Tofu, 8 oz
- Veggie burgers, 3.7 oz

# Think Thin Food Lists
## Lunch Options (Protein)

## 250-Calorie Portions

### Meat and Poultry:

- Beef brisket or corned beef brisket, 3.5 oz
- Beef, ground or hamburger, 90% lean, 3.8 oz
- Chicken, breast, 5 oz
- Chicken burger or sausage, or ground chicken, 4.4 oz
- Deli: chicken breast, ham, turkey breast, or roast beef, 6.2 oz
- Ham, sirloin steak, or veal loin, 5 oz
- Hotdog, beef, 2.5 oz
- Hotdog, beef, 97% fat-free, 5 oz **plus** ½ item from this list
- Turkey, breast, 4.7 oz
- Turkey, burger or hotdog or sausage, or ground turkey, 3.7 oz

### Dairy:

- Cheese, cottage, 1% (1⅔ cups) or 4% (1 cup)
- Cheese, farmer's, 3.3 oz
- Cheese, goat, 2.5 oz
- Cheese, hard, 2 oz
- Cheese, ricotta, fat-free (1⅔ cups) or part-skim (¾ cup)
- Eggs, 3
- Egg whites, 6½ **plus** ½ item from this list
- Milk, skim, 1¼ cups **plus** ½ item from this list
- Yogurt, plain, non-fat, ⅞ cup **plus** ½ item from this list
- Yogurt, flavored or full-fat (check label)

### Fish and Seafood:

- Calamari, crab, lobster, oysters, shrimp, or scallops, 8.2 oz
- Cod, flounder, tilapia, or sole, 7.5 oz
- Imitation crab, 8.1 oz
- Salmon, cooked, 5 oz or canned, 6.2 oz
- Salmon, smoked, 3.8 oz **plus** ½ item from this list
- Sushi (pick 2 of these 3 choices):
  - 3 pieces eel roll or California roll
  - 4 pieces tuna roll or salmon roll
  - 5.5 pieces cucumber roll
- Swordfish, 6.2 oz
- Tuna, cooked, 5 oz or chunk light canned, 8.7 oz

### Vegetarian:

- Beans or lentils, cooked, 7.5 oz
- Chili, canned (check label)
- Hummus, ½ cup plus 1 Tbsp
- Nut butters; peanut, almond, or cashew; 2½ Tbsp
- Pizza, 2.9 oz (1¼ slices of 14-inch thin-crust, plain)
- Seitan, 5.7 oz
- Tahini, 2.5 Tbsp
- Tempeh, uncooked, 4.4 oz
- Tofu, 8 oz, cooked with 1 Tbsp olive oil
- Veggie burgers, 4 oz **plus** 1 oz cheese

# Think Thin Food Lists
## Dinner Options (Protein)

### 300-Calorie Portions

**Meat and Poultry:**

- Beef brisket or corned beef brisket, 4.2 oz
- Beef, ground or hamburger, 90% lean, 4.5 oz
- Chicken, breast, 6 oz
- Chicken burger or sausage, or ground chicken, 5.2 oz
- Ham, sirloin steak, or veal loin, 6 oz
- Hotdog, beef, 3 oz
- Hotdog, beef, 97% fat-free, 6 oz **plus** ½ item from this list
- Lamb, pork chop, or roast beef, 5 oz
- Turkey, breast, 5.7 oz
- Turkey burger or hotdog or sausage, or ground turkey, 4.5 oz

**Dairy:**

- Cheese, cottage, 1% (2 cups) or 4% (1⅓ cups)
- Cheese, farmer's, 4 oz
- Cheese, goat, 3 oz
- Cheese, hard, 2.4 oz
- Eggs, 4
- Yogurt, plain, non-fat, 1⅛ cups **plus** ½ item from this list
- Yogurt, low-fat, 1 cup **plus** ½ item from this list
- Yogurt, flavored or full-fat (check label)

**Fish and Seafood:**

- Calamari, crab, lobster, oysters, shrimp, or scallops, 9.9 oz
- Cod, flounder, sole, or tilapia, 9 oz
- Imitation crab, 9.7 oz
- Salmon or tuna, cooked, 6 oz
- Sushi (pick 2 of these 3 choices):
  - 4 pieces eel roll or California roll
  - 5 pieces tuna roll or salmon roll
  - 7 pieces cucumber roll
- Swordfish, 7.5 oz

**Vegetarian:**

- Beans or lentils, cooked, 9 oz
- Burrito, commercially prepared, up to 300 calories (check label)
- Chili, canned (check label)
- Hummus, ¾ cup
- Nut butters; peanut, almond, or cashew; 3 Tbsp
- Pizza, 3.5 oz (1½ slices of 14-inch thin-crust, plain **or** 2 slices of 12-inch thin-crust, plain)
- Seitan, 6.9 oz
- Tahini, 3 Tbsp
- Tempeh, uncooked, 5.2 oz
- Tofu, 8 oz, cooked with 2 Tbsp olive oil
- Veggie burgers, 5 oz **plus** 1 oz veggie slice or soy cheese

# Think Thin Food Lists
## Starter Salad and Soup Options

You can use up to 1 tablespoon of fat-free salad dressing; it has been included in the calorie count for the salad items. If you want to use more than 1 tablespoon or another kind of salad dressing, use Add-On or Bonus Calories or use an item from the condiment list.

| Starter Salads | Starter Soups |
|---|---|
| • **All-American Salad:**<br>Combine 3 cups iceberg lettuce with ¼ cup grated carrot and 4 slices cucumber.<br><br>• Cabbage and Snow Pea Salad with Poppy Dressing (page 233)<br><br>• **Escarole or Endive Salad with Goat Cheese:**<br>Combine 3 cups escarole or endive with 1 tsp goat cheese.<br><br>• **Mixed Greens Salad:**<br>Combine 3 cups mixed greens (such as arugula, butterhead, endive, or radicchio) with ½ cup chopped vegetables.<br><br>• **Romaine Salad:**<br>Combine 3 cups romaine lettuce with 2 Tbsp plain croutons.<br><br>• **Spinach Salad:**<br>Combine 3 cups spinach greens with 7 grape tomatoes. | • Hearty Vegetable Soup, 1¼ cups (page 233)<br><br>• Commercially available soup, 50-calorie portion<br><br>• Chicken, beef, or vegetable broth, 1 cup, with up to 35 calories of choice of cooked vegetable |

# Think Thin Food Lists
## Fruit Options: 100-Calorie Portions

Fruits can be fresh or frozen (without syrup). If you prefer to eat canned fruit, make sure it is packed in water or light syrup and drained well; check label for calories. Use Bonus Calories if you would like dried fruits.

- Apple, 1 large
- Applesauce, sweetened, ½ cup
- Applesauce, unsweetened, 1 cup
- Apricots, 6 medium
- Avocado, ⅓ medium, 2 oz
- Banana, 1 medium
- Blackberries, 1½ cups
- Blueberries, 1¼ cups
- Cantaloupe, ½ medium
- Cherries, 1 cup
- Figs, 3 small
- Grapefruit, 1 large
- Grapes, 1 cup
- Honeydew melon, ¼ medium
- Kiwifruit, 2 medium
- Mango, ⅔ medium

- Nectarines, 1½ medium
- Oranges, 1½ medium
- Papaya, 1 medium
- Peaches, 2 medium
- Pear, 1 medium
- Persimmon, 1 medium
- Pineapple, 1¼ cups
- Plantain, cooked, ⅝ cup
- Plums, 3 medium
- Pomegranate, 1 medium
- Prunes, stewed, ⅓ cup
- Raspberries, 1½ cups
- Strawberries, 2 cups
- Tangerines, 2½ medium
- Watermelon, diced, 2 cups

## Think Thin Food Lists
### Vegetable Options: 50-Calorie Portions

- Artichoke, cooked, 1 small

- Artichoke hearts, canned, 8 oz

- Beans, green, Italian, string, or wax, 1¼ cups cooked

- Bean sprouts, 1½ cups raw **or** ¾ cup cooked

- Beets, ¾ cup cooked

- Broccoli, 2 cups florets raw **or** 1½ cups cooked

- Brussels sprouts, 1 cup cooked

- Cabbage, green, red or Chinese, raw or cooked, 1½ cups

- Carrots, cooked, sliced, 1 cup

- Carrots, raw, 1 cup sliced **or** 2 medium carrots **or** 13 baby carrots

- Cauliflower, florets, raw or cooked, 1½ cups

- Celery, diced, raw or cooked, 1½ cups **or** 4 stalks (8 inches)

- Cucumbers, 2 medium

- Edamame, frozen, prepared, ¼ cup

- Eggplant, cooked, 1½ cups

- Escarole, raw or cooked, 1½ cups

- Fennel, raw or cooked, 1½ cups

- Greens (chard, collards, kale, mustard, or turnip), raw or cooked, 1½ cups

- Jícama, 1 cup raw **or** 1½ cups cooked

- Kohlrabi, 1½ cups raw **or** 1 cup cooked

- Leeks, 1 cup raw **or** 1½ cups cooked

- Mushrooms, raw or cooked, 1½ cups

- Okra, raw or cooked, 1½ cups

- Onions, ¾ cup raw **or** 1½ cups cooked

- Parsnips, cooked, ½ cup

- Peas, cooked, ⅔ cup

- Peppers (green, orange, red, or yellow), 1½ cups raw **or** 1 cup cooked

- Radishes, raw or cooked, 1½ cups

- Rutabaga, ¾ cup cooked

- Scallions, 1½ cups raw **or** 1 cup cooked

- Snap peas, ¾ cup cooked

- Spinach, 3 cups raw **or** ¾ cup cooked

- Squash, acorn, cooked, 1 cup

- Squash, spaghetti, cubes, 1¼ cups cooked

- Squash, yellow, sliced, raw or cooked, 1½ cups

- Tomatoes, canned, ¾ cup

- Tomatoes, cooked, 1½ cups

- Tomatoes, raw, 1½ cups chopped **or** 16 cherry **or** 4 plum **or** 20 grape tomatoes

- Turnips, cooked, 1½ cups

- Zucchini, 2½ cups raw **or** 1⅔ cups cooked

# *Think Thin Food Lists*
## *Grain and Starch Side Dish Options*

When choosing grains, opt for the highest-fiber, most whole version possible. Select 100 percent whole-grain or fiber-added bread products and pasta, and brown or wild rice. Bread should contain at least 3g of fiber per 100-calorie slice or 2g of fiber per 45-calorie slice. You can choose 7-grain, mixed-grain, whole-wheat, rye, or pumpernickel, as long as the first ingredient uses the word *whole* and it matches (at least) the fiber recommendation above. Check labels for calorie counts.

## 100-Calorie Portions

### Bread Products
**Bread:**
- Bagel, minis, 1½
- Bread, 45 calories per slice, 2 slices
- Bread, 100 calories per slice, 1 slice
- English muffin, whole-wheat, 1
- Pita, 4-inch diameter, 100% whole-wheat, 1½
- Tortilla wraps (check label)

**Crackers:**
- Crispbread-style cracker, 2½- x 1¼-inch, 3
- Matzoh, 1 sheet
- Melba toast, 5
- Rice cracker, ¾-inch diameter, 16
- Water cracker, 1½-inch round or square, 7
- Whole-wheat cracker, 1¼-inch square, 7
- Whole-wheat cracker, reduced-fat, 1¼-inch square, 14

**Rolls:**
- Hamburger or hotdog, ¾ (1 oz)
- Potato, 2-inch square, 1¼ (1.2 oz)
- Sourdough, medium, ¾ (1.2 oz)
- Sweet roll or Hawaiian bread, small, ¾ (1 oz)
- Whole-wheat dinner roll, soft, 2-inch square, 1 (1.1 oz)

### Starches
**Beans:**
- Chickpeas, cooked, ⅓ cup
- Kidney, red, or lima beans, cooked, ½ cup
- Lentils, cooked, ⅜ cup
- White or navy beans, cooked, ⅜ cup

**Cereals, hot and cold:**
- Bran cereal, ¾ cup
- Cream of wheat, cooked with water, ⅞ cup
- Grits, cooked with water, ¾ cup
- Oatmeal, cooked with water, ⅔ cup

**Grains:**
- Barley, cooked, ¾ cup
- Bulgur, cooked, ⅔ cup
- Quinoa, cooked, ⅜ cup
- Wheat germ, dry, 3 Tbsp

**Pasta:**
- Couscous, cooked, 3 oz
- Whole-wheat, cooked, ½ cup

**Potatoes:**
- French Fries, Baked (page 250), 4 oz
- Hash browns or potato pancakes, no partially hydrogenated oil (check label)
- Idaho or white, cooked, ⅞ cup
- Sweet potato, baked, ½ cup
- Sweet Potato Fries (page 250), 4 oz

**Rice:**
- Basmati or brown, cooked, ½ cup
- Wild, cooked, ⅔ cup

**Starchy Vegetables:**
- Corn, cooked, ½ cup or 1 medium ear
- Plantain, sliced, cooked, ⅝ cup

- Squash:
  - Acorn, cooked, 2 cups
  - Butternut, cooked, 1¼ cups
  - Butternut Squash Fries (page 250), 6.7 oz
  - Pumpkin, mashed, boiled, drained, or canned, 1¼ cups
  - Spaghetti squash, cooked, 2½ cups
  - Winter squash, cooked, 2½ cups

## 150-Calorie Portions

## Bread Products
### Bread:
- Bagel, minis, 2
- Bread, 45 calories per slice, 3 slices
- Bread, 100 calories per slice, 1½ slices
- English muffin, whole-wheat, 1½
- Pita, 4-inch diameter, 100% whole-wheat, 2
- Tortilla wraps (check label)

### Crackers:
- Crispbread-style cracker, 2½- x 1¼-inch, 4½
- Matzoh, 1½ sheets
- Melba toast, 7½
- Rice cracker, ¾-inch diameter, 24
- Water cracker, 1½-inch round or square, 10½
- Whole-wheat cracker, 1¼-inch square, 10½
- Whole-wheat cracker, reduced-fat, 1¼-inch square, 21

### Rolls:
- Hamburger or hotdog, 1 (1.5 oz)
- Potato, 2-inch square, 1¾ (1.8 oz)
- Sourdough, medium, 1 (1.8 oz)
- Sweet roll or Hawaiian bread, small, 1 (1.5 oz)
- Whole-wheat dinner roll, soft, 2-inch square, 1½ (1.6 oz)

## Starches
### Beans:
- Chickpeas, cooked, ½ cup

- Kidney, red, or lima beans, cooked, ¾ cup
- Lentils, cooked, ⅝ cup
- White or navy beans, cooked, ⅝ cup

### Cereals, hot and cold:
- Bran cereal, 1⅛ cups
- Cream of wheat, cooked with water, 1¼ cups
- Grits, cooked with water, 1⅛ cups
- Oatmeal, cooked with water, 1 cup

### Grains:
- Barley, cooked, 1⅛ cups
- Bulgur, cooked, 1 cup
- Quinoa, cooked, ⅝ cup
- Wheat germ, dry, 4½ Tbsp

### Pasta:
- Couscous, cooked, 4.5 oz
- Whole-wheat, cooked, ¾ cup

### Potatoes:
- French Fries, Baked (page 250), 6 oz
- Hash browns and potato pancakes, no partially hydrogenated oil (check label)
- Idaho or white, cooked, 1¼ cups
- Sweet potato, baked, ¾ cup
- Sweet Potato Fries (page 250), 6 oz

### Rice:
- Basmati or brown, cooked, ¾ cup
- Wild, cooked, 1 cup

### Starchy Vegetables:
- Corn, cooked, ¾ cup or 1½ medium ears
- Plantain, sliced, cooked, ⅞ cup
- Squash
  - Acorn, cooked, 3 cups
  - Butternut, cooked, 1⅞ cups
  - Butternut Squash Fries (page 250), 10 oz
  - Pumpkin, mashed, boiled, drained, or canned, 1⅞ cups
  - Spaghetti squash, cooked, 3¾ cups
  - Winter squash, cooked, 3¾ cups

# Think Thin Food Lists
## Snack Options

Choose higher-protein snacks to keep you feeling full longer. See recipes on pages 251–255 for additional snacks.

| 100-Calorie Portions | 150-Calorie Portions |
|---|---|
| • Cheese, cottage, 1% (⅔ cup) or 4% (⅜ cup) | • Cheese, cottage, 1% (1 cup) or 4% (⅔ cup) |
| • Cheese, hard, 0.8 oz | • Cheese, hard, 1.2 oz |
| • Cheese stick, 1¼ sticks | • Cheese sticks, 2 |
| • Chicken, cooked, chicken sausage, or chicken meatballs, 2 oz | • Chicken, cooked, chicken sausage, or chicken meatballs, 3 oz |
| • Eggs, 1½ | • Eggs, 2 |
| • Egg whites, 5 | • Egg whites, 4 **plus** ½ item from this list |
| • Fruit, any fruit from page 220 | • Fruit, any fruit from page 220 |
| • Milk, almond, 1 cup | • Milk, almond, 1½ cups |
| • Milk, skim or soy, 1 cup | • Milk, skim or soy, 1½ cups |
| • Nut butters; peanut, almond, or cashew; 1 Tbsp | • Nut butters; peanut, almond, or cashew; 1½ Tbsp |
| • Nuts: almonds, cashews, peanuts, or pistachios, 0.6 oz | • Nuts: almonds, cashews, peanuts, or pistachios, 0.9 oz |
| • Nuts: Brazil, macadamia, pecans, or walnuts, 0.5 oz | • Nuts: Brazil, macadamia, pecans, or walnuts, 0.75 oz |
| • Protein bar, 100-calorie portion of any bar with at least 1g fiber, 5g protein, and fewer than 10g sugar | • Protein bar, any 150-calorie bar with at least 1g fiber, 5g protein, and fewer than 10g sugar |
| • Salmon, canned, 2.5 oz | • Salmon, canned, 3.7 oz |
| • Tuna, canned, 3 oz | • Tuna, canned, 5 oz |
| • Yogurt (check label) | • Yogurt (check label) |

# Think Thin Food Lists

## Condiment and Accompaniment Options

### 20-Calorie Portions

You can select one condiment or accompaniment per day. If you want more, use Bonus Calories.

- Barbeque sauce, bottled, 1 Tbsp
- Broth, canned, beef, chicken, or vegetable, 1 cup
- Cocktail sauce, 1 Tbsp
- Cocoa powder, 1½ Tbsp
- Creamer, nondairy, liquid, 2 Tbsp
- Ginger, raw, 1 oz
- Hoisin sauce, 1 tsp
- Honey, 1 tsp
- Horseradish, bottled, 2 Tbsp
- Hot pepper sauce, 3 Tbsp
- Jam or jelly, regular, 1 tsp
- Ketchup, 1 Tbsp
- Lemon or lime juice, ⅓ cup
- Milk, skim, 3 Tbsp
- Mustard, brown, 1 Tbsp
- Mustard, yellow, 2 Tbsp
- Pickle relish, 1 Tbsp
- Pickles, dill, sliced, ½ cup
- Salsa, ¼ cup
- Sour cream, fat-free, 2 Tbsp
- Soy sauce, 2 Tbsp
- Steak sauce, 2 Tbsp
- Sweet and sour sauce, 1½ Tbsp
- Tartar sauce, 1 tsp
- Teriyaki sauce, 1 Tbsp
- Vinegar, ¼ cup

- Wasabi, prepared, 1 tsp
- Whipped topping, nondairy, 1½ Tbsp
- Worcestershire sauce, 2 Tbsp
- Yogurt, plain, non-fat, 2 Tbsp

## Add-On Options

### 50-Calorie Portions

- Avocado, mashed, 4 Tbsp
- Breadcrumb Coating, Herb and (page 249), 1 Tbsp
- Butter, light, 1 Tbsp
- Butter, regular, 1½ tsp
- Cream cheese, low-fat, 2 Tbsp
- Cream cheese, regular, 1 Tbsp
- Guacamole, 2 Tbsp
- Hummus, 2 Tbsp
- Margarine, light, trans fat–free, 2 Tbsp
- Mayonnaise, light, 1 Tbsp
- Mayonnaise, regular, 1½ tsp
- Nuts, 1 Tbsp
- Oil (canola, flaxseed, olive, safflower, sunflower, or walnut), 1 tsp
- Olives, large, 10
- Salad dressing, low-fat, 1½ Tbsp
- Salad dressing, regular, 2 tsp
- Sauce, Asian Ginger (page 249), 2½ Tbsp
- Sauce, marinara, ½ cup
- Sauce, Peanut (page 248), 1¼ Tbsp
- Sauce, sweet and sour, ¼ cup
- Seeds (pumpkin, sesame, or sunflower), 1 Tbsp
- Tahini, 2 tsp
- Yogurt, plain, low-fat, ⅓ cup

# *Think Thin Food Lists*
## *Bonus Calorie Options: 150-Calorie Portions*

Use your Bonus Calories with any meals or snacks. You can spend your Bonus Calories on any food or beverage. Just be sure to check labels or use a calorie counter to get the appropriate serving size.

## Food

- Apple chips, 1.2 oz
- Bean dip, 3 Tbsp plus 6 chips
- Brownie, 1.4 oz
- Cake, any variety (check label)
- Candy, any variety (check label)
- Chocolate, any variety, 1 oz
- Cookies, any variety, 1 oz
- French fries, shoestring, 2 oz
- Frozen yogurt or other frozen treats (check label)
- Fruit, dried, apple, blueberries, cherries, cranberries, or mango, 1.5 oz
- Fruit, dried, apricots, pears, or prunes, 2 oz
- Fruit, dried, dates, peaches, or raisins, 1.7 oz
- Ice cream, full-fat, chocolate or vanilla, ¼ cup
- Nuts: almonds, cashews, peanuts, or pistachios, 1 oz
- Nuts: Brazil, macadamia, pecans, pine nuts, or walnuts, 0.7 oz
- Pasta, cooked, ¾ cup
- Pesto, 2 Tbsp
- Popcorn, microwave, 94% fat-free, 7 cups
- Potato chips, 1 oz
- Pretzels, hard or soft, 1.5 oz
- Pudding, prepared with 2% milk, ½ cup

## Beverages

### Alcohol:

- Brandy, gin, rum, tequila, vodka, or whiskey, 2 fl oz
- Beer, 12 fl oz
- Light beer, 16 fl oz
- Wine, 6 fl oz

### Juice:

- Grapefruit juice, 11 fl oz
- Grape juice, 8 fl oz
- Orange or apple juice, 11 fl oz
- Vegetable juice, 12 fl oz **plus** ½ item from this list

### Milk:

- Skim, 13 fl oz
- 2%, 10 fl oz
- 4%, 8 fl oz
- Hot chocolate (check label)

# Think Thin Food Lists
## Bonus Calorie Options: 200-Calorie Portions

### Food

- Apple chips, 1.6 oz
- Bean dip, ¼ cup plus 8 chips
- Brownie, 1.8 oz
- Cake, any variety (check label)
- Candy, any variety (check label)
- Chocolate, any variety, 1.3 oz
- Cookies, any variety, 1.3 oz
- French fries, shoestring, 2.6 oz
- Frozen yogurt or other frozen treats (check label)
- Fruit, dried, apple, blueberries, cherries, cranberries, or mango, 2 oz
- Fruit, dried, apricots, pears, or prunes, 2.6 oz
- Fruit, dried, dates, peaches, or raisins, 2.3 oz
- Ice cream, full-fat, chocolate or vanilla, ⅓ cup
- Nuts: almonds, cashews, peanuts, or pistachios, 1.3 oz
- Nuts: Brazil, macadamia, pecans, pine nuts, or walnuts, 0.9 oz
- Pasta, cooked, 1 cup
- Pesto, 2⅔ Tbsp
- Popcorn, microwave, 94% fat-free, 9 cups
- Potato chips, 1.3 oz
- Pretzels, hard or soft, 2 oz
- Pudding, prepared with 2% milk, ⅔ cup

### Beverages

**Alcohol:**

- Brandy, gin, rum, tequila, vodka, or whiskey, 2⅔ fl oz
- Beer, 16 fl oz
- Light beer, 21 fl oz
- Wine, 8 fl oz

**Juice:**

- Grapefruit juice, 15 fl oz
- Grape juice, 10 fl oz
- Orange or apple juice, 15 fl oz
- Vegetable juice, 16 fl oz **plus** ½ item from this list

**Milk:**

- Skim, 17 fl oz
- 2%, 13 fl oz
- 4%, 11 fl oz
- Hot chocolate (check label)

# chapter 11

# Think Thin Recipes

O n the following pages, you'll find recipes that correspond to the Think Thin Eating Plan options. When making any recipe:

- **Measure out the appropriate one-serving portion.** For recipes that serve more than one person, unless otherwise noted, divide the yield equally by the number of servings to make an individual portion.

- **Condiments, sauces, butter, oil, and other toppings included in recipes have been factored into the recipe's calorie count, unless otherwise noted.** You do not need to count these as Add-On Calories, Bonus Calories, or condiments. You can also add whichever herbs and spices you would like to any recipe.

- **Check the Think Thin Formulas in Chapter 10 (pages 210–214) to see which side dishes and add-ons you may include, depending on the calorie plan you are following.** For example, breakfast recipes on the 1,600-calorie plan are complete meals and do not include a side dish.

- **You'll find instructions to slice, chop, dice, and mince ingredients.** Unless otherwise noted, these instructions mean:

  - **Sliced** = thin, flat pieces

  - **Chopped** = ¼-inch-diameter irregularly shaped chunks

- **Diced** = ⅛- to ¼-inch-diameter uniformly shaped chunks

- **Minced** = chopped finely (You can use a garlic press to mince most ingredients.)

- **Use cooking spray instead of butter or oil** unless oil is called for in a recipe or unless you wish to use these fats as your Add-On Calories or Bonus Calories.

- **Use whole grains instead of refined grains whenever possible.** Choose brown or wild rice over white, whole-grain bread over white, and whole-grain pasta over refined.

- **Use the leanest cuts of meat available.**

- **Use skinless, boneless chicken.**

# Think Thin Recipes

## stage 2 recipes

## stage 4 recipes

# breakfast recipes

## Tomato-Basil Omelet with Waffle

*Serves 1.*

2   large eggs, beaten
¼   cup halved cherry tomatoes
1   to 2 tsp fresh basil (optional)
1   whole-grain frozen waffle, toasted
1   tsp maple syrup

**Heat** a nonstick skillet over medium heat. Add eggs, tomatoes, and, if desired, basil. Cook 4 to 5 minutes or until set. Use a spatula to fold 1 side of omelet on top of other side; cook 1 minute.
**Serve** with waffle and syrup.

Calories 250, Carbohydrate 23g, Protein 16g, Total Fat 12g, Saturated Fat 3g, Cholesterol 423mg, Sugar 9g, Fiber 2g

## Bell Pepper Omelet with Toast

*Serves 1.*

1   whole egg plus 2 egg whites **or**
    ⅓ cup egg substitute, whisked*
2   Tbsp chopped red bell pepper
3   Tbsp reduced-fat shredded Cheddar
    or Colby cheese*
1   slice whole-wheat toast
2   tsp all-fruit jam

**Heat** a nonstick skillet over medium heat. Add eggs, bell pepper, and cheese. Cook until set. Serve with toast and jam.
*If using egg substitute, increase cheese to 5 Tbsp.

**With eggs:** Calories 250, Carbohydrate 20g, Protein 21g, Total Fat 9g, Saturated Fat 4g, Cholesterol 222mg, Sugar 10g, Fiber 3g

**With egg substitute:** Calories 250, Carbohydrate 20g, Protein 21g, Total Fat 10g, Saturated Fat 5g, Cholesterol 21mg, Sugar 10g, Fiber 3g

## Veggie-Bacon Wrap

*Serves 1.*

| | |
|---|---|
| 2 | tsp light mayonnaise |
| 1 | (8-inch) soft whole-wheat tortilla* |
| 4 | thin slices turkey bacon, cooked |
| ½ | cup shredded romaine lettuce |
| 1 | tsp chopped red onion |

**Spread** light mayonnaise on tortilla.
**Add** bacon, lettuce, and onion. Roll
up to eat.
*About 140 calories, with at least 3g fiber.

Calories 250, Carbohydrate 28g, Protein 14g,
Total Fat 10g, Saturated Fat 2g, Cholesterol 30mg,
Sugar 4g, Fiber 4g

## Mexican Breakfast Wrap

*Serves 1.*

| | |
|---|---|
| 1 | (8-inch) soft whole-wheat tortilla* |
| ¼ | cup shredded cheese (such as Mexican blend) |
| ½ | cup shredded romaine lettuce |
| 2 | Tbsp prepared salsa |

**Fill** tortilla with cheese, fold over, and
heat in microwave at HIGH 30 seconds.
**Open** tortilla and add lettuce and salsa.
*About 140 calories, with at least 3g fiber.

Calories 250, Carbohydrate 20g, Protein 18g,
Total Fat 13g, Saturated Fat 7g, Cholesterol 36mg,
Sugar 3g, Fiber 9g

## Cinnamon Oat Muffins

*Makes 17 muffins.*

| | |
|---|---|
| 1 | cup textured vegetable protein* |
| 2 | cups rolled oats |
| 1½ | cups 1% milk |
| 1 | cup applesauce |
| 3 | large eggs |
| 1 | cup brown sugar, packed |
| 1 | tsp salt |
| 1 | tsp baking powder |
| 2 | Tbsp cinnamon |
| 1 | tsp nutmeg |
| 2 | cups whole-wheat flour |
| ½ | cup ground flaxseed |
| 1 | cup golden raisins |
| ¼ | cup mini chocolate chips |
| ¼ | cup chopped walnuts |

**Preheat** oven to 400°F. Follow package directions to reconstitute textured
vegetable protein with water. Soak rolled
oats in milk for 45 minutes. Mix textured
vegetable protein mixture and oats mixture
with applesauce, eggs, and brown sugar.
**Add** salt, baking powder, cinnamon, nut-
meg, and flour. Gently mix. Gently fold
in flaxseed, raisins, chocolate chips, and
walnuts.
**Use** paper or foil muffin holders in 2
(12-tin) muffin tins. Fill 17 tins three-
quarters full with batter.
**Bake** at 400° for 20 minutes.
*Available in health-food stores or at most
grocery stores in the cereal or organic-
foods aisle.

Per serving (1 muffin): Calories 250, Carbohydrate 44g,
Protein 9g, Total Fat 6g, Saturated Fat 1g, Cholesterol 38mg,
Sugar 21g, Fiber 6g

# Vegetable Frittata

*Serves 1.*

Cooking spray
1   baby zucchini, thinly sliced
1   medium tomato, diced
¼   cup sliced mushrooms
3   tsp minced garlic
2   eggs, beaten
2   tsp fresh or 1 tsp dried parsley
1   Tbsp shredded Cheddar cheese
1   tsp ground white pepper

**Preheat** oven to 350°F.
**Heat** an ovenproof skillet coated with cooking spray over medium heat. Add zucchini, tomato, mushrooms, and garlic. **Cook** vegetables for 4 to 5 minutes, stirring frequently, until tender. Add eggs, parsley, cheese, and pepper. Stir until eggs are cooked through.
**Bake** at 350° for 20 minutes.

Calories 250, Carbohydrate 8g, Protein 22g,
Total Fat 15g, Saturated Fat 6g, Cholesterol 453mg,
Sugar 4g, Fiber 2g

# Berry Smoothie

*Serves 1.*

3   oz silken tofu
6   Tbsp orange juice
1   cup frozen, unsweetened berries
1   cup light vanilla soy milk

**Combine** all ingredients in a blender. Blend until smooth.

Calories 250, Carbohydrate 43g, Protein 12g,
Total Fat 5g, Saturated Fat 0g, Cholesterol 0mg,
Sugar 30g, Fiber 5g

# soup & salad

## Hearty Vegetable Soup

*Serves 16.*

1 tsp extra-virgin olive oil
1 large yellow or Vidalia onion, peeled and diced
5 stalks leeks, diced
5 large carrots, peeled and chopped
1 clove garlic, minced (optional)
10 cups water
24 oz vegetable broth
1 (14.5-oz) can chopped tomatoes
2 Tbsp fresh basil, chopped
2 Tbsp fresh cilantro, chopped
4 cups baby spinach leaves (with stems removed), chopped
  Hot red pepper flakes, to taste (optional)

**Heat** oil in a large saucepan over medium heat. Add onion, leeks, carrots, and, if desired, garlic. Cook, stirring frequently, until onions are translucent, about 3 to 5 minutes.

**Add** water, broth, tomatoes, basil, cilantro, spinach, and, if desired, pepper flakes.

**Bring** to a boil; cover, reduce heat, and simmer 45 minutes. Remove from heat; serve. Store remainder in refrigerator up to 3 days or in freezer up to 3 months.

**Per serving (1¼ cups):** Calories 50, Carbohydrate 2g, Protein 2g, Total Fat 0.8g, Saturated Fat 0g, Cholesterol 0mg, Sugar 3g, Fiber 2g

## Cabbage and Snow Pea Salad with Poppy Dressing

*Serves 8.*

1½ cups shredded green cabbage
1½ cups shredded red cabbage
3 cups snow peas
2 Tbsp tahini
⅛ tsp reduced-sodium soy sauce
1½ tsp rice wine vinegar
3 Tbsp lime juice
¼ tsp salt
½ tsp lime zest
1 tsp poppy seeds
½ medium-sized hot pepper (optional)

**Place** cabbages and snow peas in a large bowl. Blend next 7 ingredients in a food processor until smooth; add pepper, if desired. Toss cabbage mixture with dressing.

**Per serving (¾ cup):** Calories 50, Carbohydrate 5g, Protein 2.5g, Total Fat 2.5g, Saturated Fat 0.5g, Cholesterol 0mg, Sugar 1g, Fiber 2g

# lunch recipes

## Salmon or Tuna Salad with Crackers

*Serves 1.*

1   (3-oz) can pink salmon **or** 1 (4-oz) can chunk light tuna canned in water, drained

1½ tsp regular mayonnaise or 1 Tbsp light mayonnaise

1   tsp chopped fresh herbs, such as dill, basil, rosemary, or flat-leaf parsley (optional)

3   (4- x 2-inch) whole-wheat crispbread crackers

**Mix** salmon or tuna, mayonnaise, and, if desired, herbs in a small bowl.
**Serve** with crackers.

**With salmon:** Calories 300, Carbohydrate 30g, Protein 26g, Total Fat 9g, Saturated Fat 1.4g, Cholesterol 72mg, Sugar 0g, Fiber 6g

**With tuna:** Calories 300, Carbohydrate 30g, Protein 32g, Total Fat 6g, Saturated Fat 1g, Cholesterol 63mg, Sugar 0g, Fiber 6g

### calorie option

**350 calories:** Add an additional ½ tsp regular mayonnaise **or** 1 tsp light mayonnaise. Add an additional 1 oz salmon **or** 1 oz tuna.

**With salmon:** Calories 350, Carbohydrate 30g, Protein 32g, Total Fat 12g, Saturated Fat 2g, Cholesterol 96mg, Sugar 0g, Fiber 6g

**With tuna:** Calories 350, Carbohydrate 30g, Protein 39g, Total Fat 8g, Saturated Fat 1g, Cholesterol 78mg, Sugar 0g, Fiber 6g

## The Simplest Pasta Salad

*Serves 1.*

⅓   cup cooked whole-wheat pasta
1   tsp shallot, finely chopped
2   tsp fresh basil or tarragon (optional)
¼   cup chopped bell pepper
½   cup chopped mixed raw vegetables
1   tsp olive oil
1   Tbsp white vinegar
⅓   cup shredded Cheddar cheese

**Toss** pasta with shallot and, if desired, basil or tarragon; add bell pepper, vegetables, oil, vinegar, and cheese.

Calories 300, Carbohydrate 23g, Protein 13g, Total Fat 17g, Saturated Fat 8.5g, Cholesterol 39mg, Sugar 8g, Fiber 3g

### calorie option

**350 calories:** Add an additional 3 Tbsp pasta and 1 Tbsp cheese.

Calories 350, Carbohydrate 29g, Protein 16g, Total Fat 20g, Saturated Fat 10g, Cholesterol 47mg, Sugar 8g, Fiber 4g

# The Big Salad

*Serves 1.*

3    cups salad greens
1    cup chopped mixed raw vegetables
½    cup shredded cheese; **or** 3 hard-cooked eggs; **or** 4 oz lean beef; **or** 5 oz skinless chicken, turkey breast, or white fish

**Toss** greens with vegetables; top as desired. Dress salad with dressing from Add-Ons List (page 225).

**With cheese:** Calories 300, Carbohydrate 15g, Protein 17g, Total Fat 19g, Saturated Fat 12g, Cholesterol 59mg, Sugar 7g, Fiber 5g

**With eggs:** Calories 300, Carbohydrate 15g, Protein 22g, Total Fat 15g, Saturated Fat 5g, Cholesterol 635mg, Sugar 8g, Fiber 5g

**With beef:** Calories 300, Carbohydrate 15g, Protein 37g, Total Fat 10g, Saturated Fat 4g, Cholesterol 79mg, Sugar 7g, Fiber 5g

**With chicken, turkey, or fish:** Calories 300, Carbohydrate 14g, Protein 47g, Total Fat 6g, Saturated Fat 1.5g, Cholesterol 120mg, Sugar 7g, Fiber 5g

## calorie option

**350 calories:** Add an additional 1½ Tbsp cheese; **or** 4 hard-cooked egg whites; **or** ¾ oz beef; **or** 1 oz chicken, turkey, or fish.

**With cheese:** Calories 350, Carbohydrate 15g, Protein 20g, Total Fat 23g, Saturated Fat 14g, Cholesterol 78mg, Sugar 7g, Fiber 5g

**With eggs:** Calories 350, Carbohydrate 17g, Protein 36g, Total Fat 16g, Saturated Fat 5g, Cholesterol 635mg, Sugar 9g, Fiber 5g

**With beef:** Calories 350, Carbohydrate 14g, Protein 44g, Total Fat 12g, Saturated Fat 5g, Cholesterol 93mg, Sugar 7g, Fiber 5g

**With chicken, turkey, or fish:** Calories 350, Carbohydrate 14g, Protein 56g, Total Fat 7g, Saturated Fat 1.9g, Cholesterol 145mg, Sugar 7g, Fiber 5g

## California Vegetarian Sandwich with Black Beans

*Serves 1.*

5    oz tofu, thinly sliced
1    serving 15-Calorie Marinade (page 248)
Cooking spray
1½   tsp Dijon or brown mustard
2    slices whole-grain bread*
½    cup alfalfa sprouts
¼    cup canned black beans, rinsed and
     drained
2    tsp balsamic vinegar
1    tsp tarragon or basil, chopped

**Marinate** tofu in marinade at least
10 minutes or overnight.
**Grill** tofu in a pan sprayed with cooking spray over medium heat until lightly
browned on all sides, about 4 minutes.
**Spread** mustard on bread; top with tofu
and sprouts.
**Serve** with side of black beans mixed
with balsamic vinegar and herbs.
*About 80 calories and 2g fiber per slice.

Calories 300, Carbohydrate 46g, Protein 18g,
Total Fat 8g, Saturated Fat 1.3g, Cholesterol 0mg,
Sugar 7g, Fiber 9g

### calorie option

**350 calories:** Add an additional 2½ Tbsp
black beans to black bean salad.

Calories 350, Carbohydrate 52g, Protein 21g,
Total Fat 8g, Saturated Fat 1.3g, Cholesterol 0mg,
Sugar 7g, Fiber 11.5g

## Grilled Cheese and Tomato Sandwich

*Serves 1.*

2    slices whole-grain bread*
½    Tbsp light, trans fat–free margarine
1    oz cheese
1    to 2 slices tomato

**Spread** bread with margarine. Add cheese
and tomato.
**Grill** sandwich in a nonstick pan over
low heat until cheese melts and bread is
lightly browned, about 3 to 4 minutes on
each side.
*About 80 calories and 2g fiber per slice.

Calories 300, Carbohydrate 41g, Protein 15g,
Total Fat 12g, Saturated Fat 6g, Cholesterol 27mg,
Sugar 9g, Fiber 5g

### calorie option

**350 calories:** Add an additional ½ oz
cheese.

Calories 350, Carbohydrate 41g, Protein 19g,
Total Fat 16g, Saturated Fat 8g, Cholesterol 40mg,
Sugar 9g, Fiber 5g

# dinner recipes

## Warm Goat Cheese and Egg Salad

*Serves 1.*

1    cup arugula
2    cups romaine **or** 3 cups mesclun
2    tsp olive oil
1    clove garlic, halved
½    tsp vinegar or lemon juice
2    (¼-inch-thick) rounds goat cheese
     (about 1 oz)
Cooking spray
2    hard-cooked eggs, peeled and halved
6    cherry tomatoes
1    Tbsp fresh parsley or dill, chopped

**Preheat** oven to 250°F.
**Combine** greens. Mix oil, garlic, and vinegar in a small jar. Let stand for 5 minutes. Remove garlic and toss with greens.
**Place** goat cheese on aluminum foil coated with cooking spray.
**Heat** goat cheese in oven at 250° for about 5 minutes until warm.
**Arrange** eggs, tomatoes, and goat cheese over greens; sprinkle with parsley.

Calories 400, Carbohydrate 13g, Protein 22g,
Total Fat 29g, Saturated Fat 10g, Cholesterol 444mg,
Sugar 4g, Fiber 4g

### calorie option

**450 calories:** Add 1 Tbsp toasted pine nuts.

Calories 450, Carbohydrate 14g, Protein 23g,
Total Fat 35g, Saturated Fat 11g, Cholesterol 444mg,
Sugar 4g, Fiber 4g

## Western Omelet

*Serves 1.*

Cooking spray
4    eggs **or** 1 cup plus 2 Tbsp egg
     substitute
¼    tsp salt
½    tsp ground black pepper
¼    cup skim milk
½    tsp onion powder (optional)
1    cup chopped mixed raw vegetables
1    oz low-sodium deli ham, cubed*

**Spray** a nonstick skillet with cooking spray and heat over medium heat.
**Whisk** eggs with salt, pepper, milk, and, if desired, onion powder. Pour into skillet and top with vegetables and ham.
**Cook,** lifting up edges as needed until egg is set.
*If using egg substitute, increase ham to 2 oz.

Calories 400, Carbohydrate 13g, Protein 35g,
Total Fat 23g, Saturated Fat 7g, Cholesterol 863mg,
Sugar 10g, Fiber 3g

### calorie option

**450 calories:** Add an additional 1 oz ham.

Calories 450, Carbohydrate 13g, Protein 4g,
Total Fat 25g, Saturated Fat 8g, Cholesterol 879mg,
Sugar 10g, Fiber 3g

## Black Bean Burrito with Tortilla Chips and Guacamole

*Serves 1.*

1    (8-inch) soft whole-wheat tortilla*
¼    cup canned black beans, rinsed
      and drained
½    medium-sized red tomato, chopped
2    Tbsp shredded cheese
2    Tbsp salsa
1    Tbsp light sour cream
10   baked tortilla chips
2    Tbsp guacamole**

**Fill** tortilla with black beans, tomato, and cheese. Roll and top with salsa and sour cream.

**Serve** with tortilla chips and guacamole.
*About 140 calories, with at least 3g fiber.
**Use 50 calories prepared guacamole from the dairy case or make your own with ⅛ of a ripe avocado, mashed, mixed with 4 Tbsp salsa.

Calories 400, Carbohydrate 57g, Protein 16g,
Total Fat 13g, Saturated Fat 4g, Cholesterol 13mg,
Sugar 2g, Fiber 6g

### calorie option

**450 calories:** Add an additional ¼ cup black beans.

Calories 450, Carbohydrate 67g, Protein 20g,
Total Fat 13g, Saturated Fat 4g, Cholesterol 13mg,
Sugar 2g, Fiber 10g

## Veggie Tacos

*Serves 1.*

2    (0.4-oz) taco shells
1    cup shredded romaine lettuce
⅞    cup kidney beans, rinsed and drained
1    cup chopped tomatoes
½    cup chopped red onion
1    Tbsp sour cream

**Preheat** oven to 200°F. Place taco shells on a baking sheet and warm in the oven for 1 to 2 minutes, if desired.
**Fill** taco shells evenly with lettuce, beans, tomatoes, and onion. Top with sour cream.

Calories 400, Carbohydrate 64g, Protein 18g,
Total Fat 7g, Saturated Fat 2g, Cholesterol 4mg,
Sugar 8g, Fiber 15g

### calorie option

**450 calories:** Add an additional 2 Tbsp shredded cheese.

Calories 450, Carbohydrate 64g, Protein 22g,
Total Fat 13g, Saturated Fat 5g, Cholesterol 23mg,
Sugar 8g, Fiber 15g

## Falafel in Pita

*Serves 1.*

1   serving falafel (2 [1-inch] falafel rounds, made from 2 Tbsp dry falafel mix)
1   tsp canola oil
¼   cucumber, minced
1   garlic clove, minced
½   cup low-fat plain yogurt
1   (6-inch) whole-wheat pita*
½   cup thinly sliced red bell pepper
3   leaves romaine lettuce
¼   medium tomato, sliced

**Follow** package directions to make falafel, using 1 tsp oil.
**Mix** cucumber, garlic, and yogurt in a small bowl; set aside.
**Fill** pita with bell pepper, lettuce, falafel, and tomato. Top with yogurt mixture.
*About 170 calories and 4g fiber.

Calories 400, Carbohydrate 64g, Protein 18g, Total Fat 10g, Saturated Fat 2g, Cholesterol 7mg, Sugar 16g, Fiber 10g

### calorie option

**450 calories:** Add an additional 1 Tbsp falafel mix and ½ tsp oil.

Calories 450, Carbohydrate 70g, Protein 20g, Total Fat 12g, Saturated Fat 2g, Cholesterol 7mg, Sugar 17g, Fiber 12g

## Macaroni and Cheese

*Serves 6.*

2   Tbsp all-purpose flour
⅓   cup skim milk
1   Tbsp light, trans fat–free margarine
1⅞  cups (7½ oz) shredded Cheddar cheese
½   cup (2 oz) shredded 2%-fat Cheddar cheese
⅛   tsp ground black pepper
12  oz uncooked whole-wheat macaroni (34 oz or 6¾ cups cooked)
2   Tbsp plain breadcrumbs

**Preheat** oven to 400°F.
**Whisk** together flour and milk in a small bowl. Heat a large saucepan over low heat. Add flour mixture; heat, stirring constantly, 2 minutes. Increase heat to medium; stir mixture constantly until thickened. Reduce heat to low. Add margarine, regular cheese, 2%-fat cheese, and pepper. Cook until smooth, about 5 minutes.
**Add** cooked macaroni and stir well to combine. Pour into an 8-inch square baking dish; sprinkle with breadcrumbs. **Bake** at 400° for 30 minutes.

Per serving (⅙ of recipe): Calories 400, Carbohydrate 48g, Protein 21g, Total Fat 16g, Saturated Fat 9g, Cholesterol 44mg, Sugar 3g, Fiber 5g

### calorie option

**450 calories:** Add an additional 2½ oz cheese; **or** add an additional 1⅝ cups regular shredded cheese and ½ cup (4 oz) 2%-fat cheese.

Per serving (⅙ of recipe): Calories 450, Carbohydrate 48g, Protein 23g, Total Fat 20g, Saturated Fat 11.5g, Cholesterol 57mg, Sugar 3g, Fiber 5g

# Spinach Lasagna

*Serves 6.*

2   cups part-skim ricotta cheese
2   Tbsp grated Parmesan cheese
1   (10-oz) package frozen chopped spinach, thawed and drained
2   garlic cloves, minced
1   Tbsp fresh, chopped, or 1 tsp dried basil
Cooking spray
6   whole-wheat lasagna noodles, uncooked
2   cups tomato sauce
3   cups shredded mozzarella cheese

**Preheat** oven to 350°F.

**Combine** ricotta, Parmesan, spinach, garlic, and basil. Spray an 8-inch square or 7- x 11-inch baking dish with cooking spray. Place 2 lasagna noodles on bottom. Cover with ⅓ of sauce, ⅓ of ricotta mixture, and ⅓ of mozzarella. Repeat layers twice, ending with mozzarella. Tightly cover with aluminum foil.

**Bake** at 350° for 50 minutes. Uncover and let stand 15 minutes before serving.

**Store** serving-size pieces in a plastic container in refrigerator up to 3 days or in freezer up to 3 months.

**Per serving (⅙ of recipe):** Calories 400, Carbohydrate 34g, Protein 29g, Total Fat 19g, Saturated Fat 11g, Cholesterol 55mg, Sugar 4g, Fiber 6g

### calorie option

**450 calories:** Add an additional ¾ cup ricotta and 2 Tbsp Parmesan.

**Per serving (⅙ of recipe):** Calories 450, Carbohydrate 35g, Protein 33g, Total Fat 22g, Saturated Fat 13g, Cholesterol 66mg, Sugar 4g, Fiber 6g

# Mediterranean Stew

*Serves 4.*

2   Tbsp olive oil
2   garlic cloves, minced
½   cup water
1   medium zucchini, cut in 1-inch cubes
1   medium eggplant, peeled and cut in 1-inch cubes
1   (15-oz) can whole tomatoes, undrained
1   Tbsp fresh, chopped, or 1½ tsp dried basil
2   (15-oz) cans vegetable broth
1   cup uncooked couscous
1   (10-oz) package frozen chopped kale, thawed and drained; **or** 1 (10-oz) package frozen chopped spinach, thawed and drained
¾   cup feta cheese, crumbled

**Heat** a large pot over low to medium heat. Add oil and garlic. Sauté for 1 minute. Add water, zucchini, and eggplant. Simmer 5 minutes, stirring occasionally.

**Add** tomatoes with liquid, basil, broth, couscous, and kale or spinach. Cover and simmer 10 minutes. Turn off heat and ladle evenly into bowls. Crumble feta cheese evenly over each serving.

**Per serving (24 oz):** Calories 400, Carbohydrate 60g, Protein 16g, Total Fat 12g, Saturated Fat 3.3g, Cholesterol 8mg, Sugar 13g, Fiber 11g

### calorie option

**450 calories:** Add an additional ½ cup plus 1 Tbsp feta cheese.

**Per serving (24 oz):** Calories 450, Carbohydrate 61g, Protein 22g, Total Fat 14g, Saturated Fat 5g, Cholesterol 13mg, Sugar 13g, Fiber 11g

## Stick-to-Your-Ribs Beef or Turkey and Potato Soup

*Serves 4.*

Cooking spray
1½ lb 90% lean ground beef **or** 1¾ lb lean ground turkey
3 cups water
1 medium Vidalia onion, peeled and chopped
½ cup chopped celery
¼ tsp salt
⅛ tsp black pepper
1 bay leaf and 2 whole cloves tied up in small piece of cheesecloth
12 oz potatoes, with skin, chopped (2¼ cups)
½ cup chopped carrots
2 Tbsp fresh parsley, chopped

**Coat** a large saucepan with cooking spray; heat over medium heat. Add beef or turkey, breaking into small chunks. Cook throughly, about 10 to 12 minutes. Add water, onion, celery, salt, pepper, and cheesecloth bag. Bring to a boil; reduce heat to simmer. Add potatoes, carrots, and parsley.
**Simmer** 30 minutes. Remove and discard cheesecloth bag.

**Per serving (17 oz):** Calories 400, Carbohydrate 21g, Protein 37g, Total Fat 17g, Saturated Fat 7g, Cholesterol 111mg, Sugar 3g, Fiber 3g

### calorie option

**450 calories:** Add an additional 4.8 oz beef or 6 oz turkey.

**Per serving (17 oz):** Calories 450, Carbohydrate 21g, Protein 42g, Total Fat 20g, Saturated Fat 8g, Cholesterol 129mg, Sugar 3g, Fiber 3g

## Mom's Meatloaf

*Serves 4.*

1 lb 90% lean ground beef **or** 1¼ lb lean ground turkey
1 whole egg
1 medium-sized white onion, peeled and chopped
1 cup skim milk
1 cup plain breadcrumbs
⅛ tsp salt
⅛ tsp black pepper
1 tsp Worcestershire sauce (optional)
Garlic powder, to taste (optional)
Cooking spray
2 Tbsp brown sugar
1 Tbsp yellow mustard
¼ cup ketchup

**Preheat** oven to 350°F.
**Combine** first 7 ingredients; if desired, add Worcestershire sauce and garlic powder. Form into a loaf; place on baking sheet coated with cooking spray.
**Combine** brown sugar, mustard, and ketchup in a separate bowl. Pour over loaf.
**Bake** at 350° for 55 minutes.

**Per serving with beef (¼ of recipe):** Calories 400, Carbohydrate 34g, Protein 31g, Total Fat 14g, Saturated Fat 5g, Cholesterol 128mg, Sugar 14g, Fiber 2g

**Per serving with turkey (¼ of recipe):** Calories 400, Carbohydrate 34g, Protein 37g, Total Fat 13g, Saturated Fat 3g, Cholesterol 154mg, Sugar 14g, Fiber 2g

### calorie option

**450 calories:** Add an additional 4 oz beef or 4 oz ground turkey (for total of 24 oz or 1½ lb).

**Per serving with beef (¼ of recipe):** Calories 450, Carbohydrate 34g, Protein 36g, Total Fat 17g, Saturated Fat 6.5g, Cholesterol 146mg, Sugar 14g, Fiber 2g

# Quick-and-Easy Chili

*Serves 4.*

1   tsp canola oil
1   cup chopped green bell pepper
½   cup chopped white onion
2   minced garlic cloves (about 2 tsp)
2   (5-oz) cans chicken breast meat, rinsed and drained; **or** 10 oz cooked chicken breast, chopped*
1   cup chicken broth
1   (15-oz) can Great Northern or white beans, rinsed and drained
1   (15-oz) can black beans, rinsed and drained
1   (15-oz) can chopped tomatoes, undrained
1   cup tomato sauce
2   Tbsp balsamic vinegar
½   tsp ground cumin
1   Tbsp chili powder

**Heat** a large saucepan over medium heat. Add oil, bell pepper, onion, garlic, and chicken. Reduce heat to low. Add broth; simmer 3 minutes. Add Great Northern beans, black beans, and tomatoes with liquid. Simmer for 5 minutes. Add tomato sauce, vinegar, cumin, and chili powder. Stir well and simmer for 5 more minutes.
*If making vegetarian chili, leave out chicken and add 5 oz more Great Northern or black beans, and use vegetable broth instead of chicken broth.

Per serving (24 oz): Calories 400, Carbohydrate 65g, Protein 29g, Total Fat 5g, Saturated Fat 0.8g, Cholesterol 18mg, Sugar 13g, Fiber 17g

## calorie option

**450 calories:** Add an additional 2 cans chicken or an additional 10 oz cooked chicken. If making vegetarian chili, add an additional 10 oz Great Northern or black beans.

Per serving (24 oz): Calories 450, Carbohydrate 65g, Protein 39g, Total Fat 6g, Saturated Fat 1g, Cholesterol 35mg, Sugar 14g, Fiber 17g

# Slow-Cooked Steak with Brown Rice

*Serves 4.*

1   (12-oz) round sirloin or flank steak, cut in 1-inch cubes*
1   cup uncooked brown rice
1¾  cups reduced-fat, reduced-sodium cream of mushroom soup
2   cups water
1   cup sliced mushrooms
4   medium carrots, chopped

**Combine** steak with rice, soup, water, mushrooms, and carrots in a 5-, 6-, or 7-qt slow cooker. Mix well, cover, and cook on LOW for 7 to 8 hours.
*No more than 160 calories and 2g saturated fat per 4-oz serving.

Per serving (¼ of recipe): Calories 400, Carbohydrate 51g, Protein 25g, Total Fat 10g, Saturated Fat 3g, Cholesterol 48mg, Sugar 6g, Fiber 5g

## calorie option

**450 calories:** Add an additional 4 oz steak.

Per serving (¼ of recipe): Calories 450, Carbohydrate 52g, Protein 30g, Total Fat 11g, Saturated Fat 3.7g, Cholesterol 63mg, Sugar 6g, Fiber 5g

# Asian Beef and Broccoli Stir-Fry

*Serves 4.*

### Marinade Ingredients:
½ cup rice vinegar
3 Tbsp sesame oil
2 Tbsp lemon juice

### Stir-Fry Ingredients:
1 (1-lb, 6-oz) beef tenderloin, sliced in thin strips*
Cooking spray
8 cups broccoli florets
3 Tbsp minced garlic
1½ Tbsp minced ginger

**Mix** marinade ingredients and place in a shallow dish. Add meat and marinate at room temperature at least 15 minutes or in refrigerator up to 4 hours.

**Preheat** a large nonstick skillet over medium heat. Coat pan with cooking spray.

**Remove** beef from marinade; discard remaining marinade. Cook beef until browned, about 8 to 10 minutes, turning once or twice.

**Remove** beef from pan; set aside. Add broccoli to pan. Cook 4 to 5 minutes until desired tenderness, stirring often. Add garlic and ginger, stirring to prevent burning. Combine broccoli and beef mixture to warm through.

*No more than 230 calories and 12g of fat per 5-oz serving.

Per serving (¼ of recipe): Calories 400, Carbohydrate 15g, Protein 40g, Total Fat 19g, Saturated Fat 5g, Cholesterol 83mg, Sugar 3g, Fiber 5g

## calorie option

**450 calories:** Add an additional 6 oz beef.

Per serving (¼ of recipe): Calories 450, Carbohydrate 15g, Protein 49g, Total Fat 21g, Saturated Fat 6g, Cholesterol 106mg, Sugar 3g, Fiber 5g

# Greek-Style Couscous with Grilled Chicken

*Serves 4.*

3 garlic cloves, minced
1 Tbsp plus 1 tsp olive oil
1½ cups cooked couscous (¾ cup uncooked)
¼ cup Parmesan cheese
2 tsp fresh or 1 tsp dried basil
⅓ cup sliced black olives
1 (15-oz) can stewed tomatoes, drained
14 oz grilled chicken breast

**Heat** a small pan over medium heat. Sauté garlic in oil 2 to 3 minutes. Stir in cooked couscous. Stir in cheese, basil, olives, and tomatoes, or sprinkle over top before serving. Cook 2 minutes, stirring constantly.

**Serve** topped with grilled chicken.

Per serving (¼ of recipe): Calories 400, Carbohydrate 35g, Protein 39g, Total Fat 11g, Saturated Fat 3g, Cholesterol 88mg, Sugar 5g, Fiber 3g

## calorie option

**450 calories:** Add an additional 4 oz chicken.

Per serving (¼ of recipe): Calories 450, Carbohydrate 35g, Protein 48g, Total Fat 12g, Saturated Fat 3g, Cholesterol 113mg, Sugar 5g, Fiber 3g

# Sizzling Stir-Fry

*Serves 1.*

1   Tbsp canola or sesame oil
5   oz skinless, boneless chicken breast, sliced in thin strips; **or** 3½ oz beef tenderloin; **or** 6½ oz shrimp (deveined and tails removed); **or** 7 oz tofu, cut in 2-inch cubes
½   cup sliced bell pepper; **or** ½ cup frozen broccoli florets, cauliflower florets, or sliced carrots
½   cup shelled edamame
2   tsp reduced-sodium soy sauce

**Heat** oil in a nonstick skillet over medium heat. Add chicken, beef, shrimp, or tofu. Cook through (about 10 to 12 minutes for chicken or beef, 3 minutes for shrimp, or 6 to 7 minutes for tofu). Set aside.
**Add** desired vegetable and edamame to skillet; cook 6 to 7 minutes, stirring often. Stir in soy sauce; add chicken, beef, shrimp, or tofu. Continue heating until thoroughly warmed.

Calories 400, Carbohydrate 13g, Protein 44g,
Total Fat 19g, Saturated Fat 2.5g, Cholesterol 82mg
(215mg for shrimp), Sugar 3g, Fiber 6g

## calorie option

**450 calories:** Add an addtional 1 oz chicken, 1 oz beef, 1½ oz shrimp, or 2 oz tofu.

Calories 450, Carbohydrate 22g, Protein 47g,
Total Fat 20g, Saturated Fat 3g, Cholesterol 280mg,
Sugar 8g, Fiber 8g

# Spaghetti and Meatballs

*Serves 1.*

¾   cup cooked whole-grain pasta (⅜ cup uncooked)
3   (1-oz) cooked turkey meatballs*
½   cup tomato sauce
1   Tbsp Parmesan cheese

**Mix** cooked pasta with meatballs and sauce. Microwave at HIGH about 1 minute to warm to desired temperature.
**Top** with cheese before serving.
*Purchase prepared turkey meatballs. Or make your own by mixing 4 oz lean ground turkey with 1 Tbsp seasoned breadcrumbs and ½ tsp each dried basil, oregano, and rosemary (or 1 tsp each if using fresh herbs); or use 4 oz seasoned lean ground turkey. Form into balls. Coat a skillet with cooking spray and heat over medium heat. Place meatballs in pan; heat for 7 to 9 minutes, turning occasionally to cook through.

Calories 400, Carbohydrate 43g, Protein 34g,
Total Fat 11g, Saturated Fat 3g, Cholesterol 74mg,
Sugar 1g, Fiber 7g

## calorie option

**450 calories:** Add an additional meatball.

Calories 450, Carbohydrate 43g, Protein 42g,
Total Fat 14g, Saturated Fat 4g, Cholesterol 97mg,
Sugar 1g, Fiber 7g

# Slow-Cooked Lamb

*Serves 4.*

1   cup sliced potatoes, with skin
1   (1-lb) boneless lamb loin, cut in 1-inch cubes
1   Vidalia or yellow onion, peeled and diced
¼   tsp salt
½   tsp black pepper
½   tsp ground cumin
1   lb zucchini, sliced
6   oz frozen artichoke hearts, thawed and halved; **or** 6 oz artichoke hearts jarred in brine*
2   cups diced tomatoes
2   cups water

**Place** sliced potatoes in bottom of a 5-qt slow cooker. Add remaining ingredients in the order listed.

**Cover** and cook on LOW 8 to 10 hours. Stir before serving.

*Be careful not to purchase jarred marinated artichoke hearts, as these contain four times more calories.

**Per serving (¼ of recipe):** Calories 400, Carbohydrate 27g, Protein 27g, Total Fat 22g, Saturated Fat 9g, Cholesterol 79mg, Sugar 6g, Fiber 7g

## calorie option

**450 calories:** Add an additional 3 oz lamb.

**Per serving (¼ of recipe):** Calories 450, Carbohydrate 27g, Protein 29g, Total Fat 26g, Saturated Fat 11g, Cholesterol 94mg, Sugar 6g, Fiber 7g

# Barbeque Pork and Rice

*Serves 4.*

2   Tbsp canola oil
¾   cup white onion, chopped
2   Tbsp Worcestershire sauce
16  oz lean ground pork tenderloin
½   cup chicken broth
¼   cup barbeque sauce
1   (28-oz) can crushed tomatoes, undrained
1   cup cooked wild or brown rice

**Heat** oil in a large saucepan over medium heat. Add onion and sauté 2 minutes. Lower heat to medium-low. **Add** Worcestershire sauce; cover and cook 5 minutes. Uncover; add pork and broth. Cook 4 minutes, stirring frequently. Add barbeque sauce and tomatoes with liquid.

**Cover** saucepan and continue to simmer until pork is thoroughly cooked.

**Divide** evenly into 4 bowls. Add ¼ cup cooked rice to each bowl and top with ¼ of pork.

**Per serving (¼ of recipe):** Calories 400, Carbohydrate 51g, Protein 30g, Total Fat 11g, Saturated Fat 1.6g, Cholesterol 74mg, Sugar 7g, Fiber 6g

## calorie option

**450 calories:** Add an additional 6 oz pork.

**Per serving (¼ of recipe):** Calories 450, Carbohydrate 48g, Protein 39g, Total Fat 12g, Saturated Fat 1.8g, Cholesterol 101mg, Sugar 7g, Fiber 6g

## Pork Tenderloin with Barley

*Serves 1.*

⅞  cup (4.7 oz) cooked barley (prepared according to package directions)
1   (4-oz) pork tenderloin
1   serving Herb and Breadcrumb Coating (page 249)
Cooking spray
1   cup snow peas, steamed
1   tsp olive oil
1   tsp fresh basil (optional)

**Moisten** tenderloin with water. Place crumb coating and pork in a plastic bag; shake until tenderloin is well coated.
**Coat** a pan with cooking spray. Heat over medium heat. Cook pork on both sides until cooked through, about 6 to 8 minutes. Serve with snow peas and barley mixed with oil and, if desired, basil.

Calories 400, Carbohydrate 44g, Protein 35g,
Total Fat 7g, Saturated Fat 1.6g, Cholesterol 63mg,
Sugar 0g, Fiber 12g

### calorie option

**450 calories:** Add an additional 2 oz pork.

Calories 450, Carbohydrate 44g, Protein 48g,
Total Fat 8g, Saturated Fat 2g, Cholesterol 95mg,
Sugar 0g, Fiber 12g

## Slow-Cooked Pork Tenderloin

*Serves 1.*

1   (5-oz) pork tenderloin, cut in 1-inch cubes
¼   cup uncooked quick-cooking barley
¾   cup reduced-fat, reduced-sodium cream of mushroom soup
½   cup water
½   cup pea pods
½   cup chopped celery

**Combine** pork with barley, soup, water, pea pods, and celery in a 1½-qt slow cooker. Mix well, cover, and cook on LOW 5 to 6 hours.

Calories 400, Carbohydrate 44g, Protein 36g,
Total Fat 9g, Saturated Fat 3g, Cholesterol 99mg,
Sugar 5g, Fiber 5g

### calorie option

**450 calories:** Add an additional 1½ oz pork.

Calories 450, Carbohydrate 44g, Protein 45g,
Total Fat 10g, Saturated Fat 3g, Cholesterol 127mg,
Sugar 5g, Fiber 5g

## Delicious Dill Fish with Fresh Asparagus

*Serves 1.*

8   small spears asparagus
1   (8-oz) boneless fish fillet (trout, snapper, or flounder)
1   tsp olive oil
⅛   tsp salt
⅛   tsp pepper
2   tsp fresh dill, chopped
2   tsp lemon juice
2   tsp capers

**Preheat** oven to 350°F.
**Blanch** asparagus 1 to 2 minutes.
**Place** fish on a sheet of aluminum foil big enough to wrap entire fillet. Drizzle fish with oil; sprinkle with salt, pepper, and dill. Arrange asparagus spears to side of fish; sprinkle fish and asparagus with lemon juice, and top with capers. Wrap loosely.
**Bake** at 350° for 12 minutes.

Calories 400, Carbohydrate 7g, Protein 50g, Total Fat 17g, Saturated Fat 4g, Cholesterol 134mg, Sugar 2g, Fiber 3g

### calorie option

**450 calories:** Add an additional 1 oz fish and ½ tsp oil.

Calories 450, Carbohydrate 7g, Protein 56g, Total Fat 21g, Saturated Fat 5g, Cholesterol 151mg, Sugar 2g, Fiber 3g

## Tilapia and Baby Greens Salad

*Serves 4.*

1   (36-oz) tilapia fillet, cut in 4 equal pieces
Cooking spray
1   avocado, sliced
¼   cup lime juice
3   Tbsp olive oil
¾   tsp salt
½   cup fresh Italian parsley or cilantro
2   Tbsp red onion, peeled and chopped
12  cups baby salad greens

**Preheat** oven to 375°F. Bring fish to room temperature.
**Heat** a large ovenproof skillet over medium heat. Spray fish with cooking spray. Place fish in skillet and cook until browned on 1 side, about 3 to 4 minutes. Turn over. Transfer skillet to oven.
**Bake** at 375° just until fish looks translucent and starts to flake (it will taste better if not overcooked), about 3 to 7 minutes, depending on thickness of fish.
**Combine** avocado with lime juice, oil, salt, parsley or cilantro, and onion.
**Gently** toss salad greens with avocado mixture and divide evenly on 4 plates. Top with fish and serve.

Per serving (¼ of recipe): Calories 400, Carbohydrate 9g, Protein 48g, Total Fat 17g, Saturated Fat 2.5g, Cholesterol 110mg, Sugar 1g, Fiber 5g

### calorie option

**450 calories:** Add an additional 12 oz fish.

Per serving (¼ of recipe): Calories 450, Carbohydrate 9g, Protein 64g, Total Fat 17g, Saturated Fat 3g, Cholesterol 146mg, Sugar 1g, Fiber 5g

# sauces & coatings

Use Add-On Calories or Bonus Calories for these sauces and coatings (with the exception of the 15-Calorie Marinade, which counts as a condiment) on chicken, fish, and other dishes. Please note that if any recipe in Chapter 11 calls for a sauce or coating, it has already been calculated into that recipe's calorie count.

## 15-Calorie Marinade

*Serves 12 or makes 24 Tbsp.*

*Use this marinade with lean chicken, pork, fish, lamb, shellfish, or steak to add flavor with just a few calories (counting it as one of your condiments). Marinate protein foods in a shallow dish or zip-top bag. Marinate tofu 10 minutes, fish no longer than 20 minutes, and other types of protein at least 30 minutes (up to overnight in the refrigerator). Discard used marinade before cooking. Save the remaining marinade in a covered container in the refrigerator up to three days or measure 2 Tbsp marinade into each section of an ice-cube tray and freeze up to a month.*

| | |
|---|---|
| 2 | fresh plums or 2 fresh apricots, sliced and pitted |
| ½ | peeled Vidalia onion |
| ½ | cup white vinegar |
| ¼ | cup balsamic vinegar |
| 1 | garlic clove, peeled |
| 1 | shallot, peeled |
| ¼ | tsp salt |
| ½ | tsp ground white or black pepper |

**Puree** all ingredients in a food processor until smooth.

Per serving (2 Tbsp): Calories 15, Carbohydrate 3g, Protein 0g, Total Fat 0g, Saturated Fat 0g, Cholesterol 0g, Sugar 4g, Fiber 0g

**Variation:** For an Asian flair, prepare marinade without vinegars and substitute ¼ cup reduced-sodium soy sauce and ½ cup rice vinegar.

Per serving (2 Tbsp): Calories 15, Carbohydrate 3g, Protein 0g, Total Fat 0g, Saturated Fat 0g, Cholesterol 0mg, Sugar 1g, Fiber 0g

## Peanut Sauce

*Serves 8.*

| | |
|---|---|
| ¼ | cup creamy peanut butter |
| 1 | Tbsp sugar |
| 2 | Tbsp hoisin sauce |
| 1 | Tbsp reduced-sodium soy sauce |
| 1 | garlic clove, minced |
| 1 | tsp sesame oil |
| 2 | tsp lime juice |
| 3 | Tbsp water |

**Combine** all ingredients in a medium mixing bowl. Stir until smooth.

Per serving (¾ oz or 1½ Tbsp): Calories 65, Carbohydrate 4g, Protein 2.3g, Total Fat 5g, Saturated Fat 1g, Cholesterol 0mg, Sugar 2g, Fiber 0.6g

## Asian Ginger Sauce

*Serves 4.*

2    Tbsp reduced-sodium soy sauce
¼    cup red wine vinegar
2    tsp minced ginger
1    Tbsp sesame oil
1    Tbsp brown sugar
2    scallions, thinly sliced

**Combine** soy sauce, vinegar, ginger, and oil in a small bowl. Set aside.

**Melt** brown sugar in a small saucepan over high heat, stirring constantly, until just melted but not burned, about 1 minute. Add soy sauce mixture. Bring to a boil until brown sugar is melted again (it will harden after you add the soy sauce mixture, but keep stirring and it will soften).

**Remove** from heat, pour into serving dish, and add scallions.

**Per serving (1.3 oz or 2½ Tbsp):** Calories 50, Carbohydrate 3.5g, Protein 0.6g, Total Fat 0.6g, Saturated Fat 0.5g, Cholesterol 0mg, Sugar 2g, Fiber 0g

## Herb and Breadcrumb Coating

*Serves 12.*

½    cup all-purpose flour
1    tsp cornstarch
1    tsp paprika
½    tsp salt
1    tsp sugar
5    tsp canola oil
1    tsp dried basil
1    tsp dried rosemary
1    Tbsp dried parsley
1    cup plain breadcrumbs

**Combine** all ingredients and mix well. Store unused coating in a zip-top bag in the freezer.

**Per serving (1 Tbsp):** Calories 65, Carbohydrate 10g, Protein 2g, Total Fat 2g, Saturated Fat 0g, Cholesterol 0mg, Sugar 1g, Fiber 1g

# starch side dishes

## Butternut Squash Fries

*Serves 3.*

Cooking spray
1   medium butternut squash, peeled, halved lengthwise, and seeded (about 1¼ lb)*
1   tsp kosher or table salt

**Preheat** oven to 450°F.
**Coat** a baking sheet with cooking spray.
**Cut** squash in ½- to ¾-inch sticks, arrange on baking sheet, and sprinkle with salt.
**Bake** at 450° for 40 minutes. Use a spatula to turn fries halfway through baking. Fries are done when edges are crispy.
*Total weight after seeding. Alternatively, you may use 1¼ lb packaged peeled and cubed squash.

**Per serving (6½ oz):** Calories 100, Carbohydrate 22g, Protein 2g, Total Fat 0g, Saturated Fat 0g, Cholesterol 0mg, Sugar 4g, Fiber 4g

## Baked French Fries

*Serves 4.*

Cooking spray
1   lb baking potatoes
1   tsp kosher or table salt

**Preheat** oven to 450°F.
**Coat** a baking sheet with cooking spray.
Peel potatoes and cut in ½- to ¾-inch sticks; sprinkle with salt.
**Bake** at 450° for 40 minutes. Use a spatula to turn fries halfway through baking. Fries are done when edges are crispy.

**Per serving (4 oz):** Calories 100, Carbohydrate 21g, Protein 2.5g, Total Fat 0g, Saturated Fat 0g, Cholesterol 0mg, Sugar 1g, Fiber 1.5g

## Sweet Potato Fries

*Serves 4.*

Cooking spray
1   lb sweet potatoes, peeled
1   tsp kosher or table salt

**Preheat** oven to 450°F.
**Coat** a baking sheet with cooking spray.
Cut sweet potato in ½- to ¾-inch sticks and sprinkle with salt.
**Bake** at 450° for 40 minutes. Use a spatula to turn fries halfway through baking. Fries are done when edges are crispy.

**Per serving (4 oz):** Calories 100, Carbohydrate 23g, Protein 2g, Total Fat 0g, Saturated Fat 0g, Cholesterol 0mg, Sugar 5g, Fiber 3.4g

# snack recipes

## Mixed Berry Smoothie

*Serves 1.*

½   cup frozen, unsweetened mixed
     berries
½   cup plain soy milk, skim milk, or
     enriched rice or almond milk
¼   tsp vanilla extract

**Combine** all ingredients in a blender.
Blend until smooth.

Calories 100, Carbohydrate 14g, Protein 4g,
Total Fat 3g, Saturated Fat 0g, Cholesterol 0mg,
Sugar 10g, Fiber 3g

### calorie option

**150 calories:** Blend ⅔ cup of any variety of
frozen berries with ⅔ cup plain soy milk, skim
milk, or enriched rice or almond milk; add
¼ tsp vanilla extract.

Calories 150, Carbohydrate 18g, Protein 5g,
Total Fat 3g, Saturated Fat 0g, Cholesterol 0mg,
Sugar 13g, Fiber 4g

## Cannoli-Style Cereal

*Serves 1.*

3   Tbsp high-fiber cereal
3   Tbsp fat-free ricotta cheese
1   tsp walnuts, chopped
1   tsp mini chocolate chip morsels

**Layer** cereal, ricotta cheese, chopped
walnuts, and chocolate chip morsels in
a bowl. Serve immediatetly.

Calories 100, Carbohydrate 17g, Protein 5g,
Total Fat 3g, Saturated Fat 1g, Cholesterol 8mg,
Sugar 4g, Fiber 6g

### calorie option

**150 calories:** Layer ¼ cup high-fiber cereal,
¼ cup fat-free ricotta cheese, 1 tsp chopped
walnuts, and 1 tsp mini chocolate chips.

Calories 150, Carbohydrate 21g, Protein 7g,
Total Fat 3g, Saturated Fat 1g, Cholesterol 10mg,
Sugar 5g, Fiber 7g

# Cheese Roll-Up

*Serves 1.*

2   slices soy cheese*
1   tsp slivered almonds, toasted
1   tsp dried fruit (such as raisins or
    blueberries)

**Place** cheese slices on a flat surface; sprinkle each slice with ½ tsp almonds and ½ tsp dried fruit. Roll up to eat. *No more than 40 calories and 2g fat per slice, with at least 200mg calcium.

Calories 100, Carbohydrate 4g, Protein 9g,
Total Fat 6g, Saturated Fat 0g, Cholesterol 0mg,
Sugar 2g, Fiber 0g

## calorie option

**150 calories:** Sprinkle 2 cheese slices with 2 tsp (4.6g) toasted slivered almonds and 2 tsp dried fruit, such as raisins or blueberries. Roll up to eat.

Calories 150, Carbohydrate 7g, Protein 9g,
Total Fat 7g, Saturated Fat 0g, Cholesterol 0mg,
Sugar 4g, Fiber 1g

# Chocolaty Yogurt

*Serves 1.*

4   oz low-fat plain yogurt
1   tsp honey or agave nectar
6   chocolate chip morsels

**Combine** all ingredients in a small bowl. Serve immediately, or cover and chill until ready to serve.

Calories 100, Carbohydrate 17g, Protein 6g,
Total Fat 3g, Saturated Fat 2g, Cholesterol 7mg,
Sugar 16g, Fiber 0g

## calorie option

**150 calories:** Combine 6 oz low-fat plain yogurt with ½ tsp honey or agave nectar, 1 tsp mini chocolate chip morsels, and ⅓ cup raspberries.

Calories 150, Carbohydrate 23g, Protein 10g,
Total Fat 4g, Saturated Fat 3g, Cholesterol 10mg,
Sugar 20g, Fiber 3g

# Nut Butter on Fruit

*Serves 1.*

½ medium apple or pear
1½ tsp peanut, cashew, or almond butter

**Cut** apple or pear in 3 slices. Spread each slice with ½ tsp peanut, cashew, or almond butter.

Calories 100, Carbohydrate 14g, Protein 2g,
Total Fat 4g, Saturated Fat 1g, Cholesterol 0mg,
Sugar 10.2g, Fiber 3g

## calorie option

**150 calories:** Cut one medium apple or pear in 6 slices. Spread slices evenly with 3 tsp peanut, cashew, or almond butter.

Calories 150, Carbohydrate 26g, Protein 4g,
Total Fat 8g, Saturated Fat 2g, Cholesterol 0mg,
Sugar 19g, Fiber 5g

# Sweet Sesame Cracker

*Serves 1.*

2 (2½-inch) graham cracker squares
1 tsp tahini sauce
1 tsp toasted sesame seeds

**Spread** 1 graham cracker square with tahini sauce; sprinkle with sesame seeds. Top with remaining graham cracker square.

Calories 100, Carbohydrate 13g, Protein 2g,
Total Fat 6g, Saturated Fat 1g, Cholesterol 0mg,
Sugar 5g, Fiber 1g

## calorie option

**150 calories:** Spread 1 graham cracker square with 1 Tbsp tahini sauce; sprinkle with sesame seeds. Top with remaining graham cracker square.

Calories 150, Carbohydrate 15g, Protein 4g,
Total Fat 11g, Saturated Fat 2g, Cholesterol 0mg,
Sugar 6g, Fiber 2g

# Tomato-Basil Cheesy Crackers

*Serves 1.*

3   whole-wheat crackers*
1   slice soy cheese**
6   cherry tomatoes, halved
Chopped fresh basil

**Top** each cracker with ⅓ slice cheese. Place in toaster oven at 200°F for 1 minute or in microwave on HIGH 30 seconds until cheese melts. Top each cracker evenly with cherry tomato halves and sprinkle with chopped fresh basil.
**No more than 40 total calories, with at least 2g fiber per cracker.
**No more than 40 calories and 2g fat, with at least 200mg calcium.

Calories 100, Carbohydrate 10g, Protein 6g,
Total Fat 4g, Saturated Fat 0g, Cholesterol 0mg,
Sugar 3g, Fiber 2g

### calorie option

**150 calories:** Top 6 whole-wheat crackers each with ⅓ slice soy cheese (using 2 slices total). Top crackers evenly with 9 cherry tomatoes, halved, and chopped fresh basil.

Calories 150, Carbohydrate 16g, Protein 7g,
Total Fat 7g, Saturated Fat 1g, Cholesterol 0mg,
Sugar 3g, Fiber 2g

# Veggies and Hummus

*Serves 1.*

¾   cup mixed raw vegetables
3   Tbsp hummus

**Chop** vegetables into bite-sized pieces. Serve with hummus for dipping.

Calories 100, Carbohydrate 12g, Protein 5g,
Total Fat 5g, Saturated Fat 0g, Cholesterol 0mg,
Sugar 2g, Fiber 5g

### calorie option

**150 calories:** Serve ¾ cup mixed raw vegetables, chopped into bite-sized pieces, with 5 Tbsp hummus.

Calories 150, Carbohydrate 16g, Protein 8g,
Total Fat 7g, Saturated Fat 1g, Cholesterol 0mg,
Sugar 2g, Fiber 7g

# Veggies and Salsa

*Serves 1.*

2   cups mixed raw vegetables
5   Tbsp salsa

**Chop** vegetables into bite-sized pieces. Serve with salsa for dipping.

Calories 100, Carbohydrate 20g, Protein 6g,
Total Fat 0g, Saturated Fat 0g, Cholesterol 0mg,
Sugar 9g, Fiber 7g

### calorie option

**150 calories:** Serve 1½ cups mixed raw vegetables, chopped into bite-sized pieces, with 4 Tbsp salsa and 1 stick string cheese.

Calories 150, Carbohydrate 17g, Protein 11g,
Total Fat 7g, Saturated Fat 3.5g, Cholesterol 20mg,
Sugar 7g, Fiber 5g

# Veggies and Guacamole

*Serves 1.*

1   cup mixed raw vegetables
2⅓ Tbsp guacamole

**Chop** vegetables into bite-sized pieces.
Serve with guacamole for dipping.

Calories 100, Carbohydrate 11g, Protein 3g,
Total Fat 6g, Saturated Fat 3g, Cholesterol 0mg,
Sugar 4g, Fiber 3g

## calorie option

**150 calories:** Serve 1½ cups mixed raw
vegetables, chopped into bite-sized pieces,
with 4 Tbsp guacamole.

Calories 150, Carbohydrate 18g, Protein 5g,
Total Fat 10g, Saturated Fat 5g, Cholesterol 0mg,
Sugar 7g, Fiber 4g

# Veggies and Peanut Sauce

*Serves 1.*

1   cup mixed raw vegetables
1½ Tbsp Peanut Sauce (page 248)

**Chop** vegetables into bite-sized pieces.
Serve with sauce for dipping.

Calories 100, Carbohydrate 12g, Protein 4g,
Total Fat 5g, Saturated Fat 1g, Cholesterol 0mg,
Sugar 4g, Fiber 3g

## calorie option

**150 calories:** Serve 1½ cups mixed raw
vegetables, chopped into bite-sized pieces,
with 2 Tbsp Peanut Sauce.

Calories 150, Carbohydrate 17g, Protein 6g,
Total Fat 7g, Saturated Fat 1g, Cholesterol 0mg,
Sugar 7g, Fiber 5g

# lunch recipes

## Barbeque Chicken Salad

*Serves 1.*

| | |
|---|---|
| 4 | oz cooked chicken breast, cut in strips |
| ½ | cup cooked corn |
| ½ | cup low-fat plain yogurt |
| 1 | Tbsp barbeque sauce |
| 1 | tsp white vinegar |
| 3 | cups shredded romaine lettuce |

**Combine** first 5 ingredients in a bowl. Spoon over bed of lettuce.

Calories 300, Carbohydrate 43g, Protein 40g, Total Fat 4g, Saturated Fat 2g, Cholesterol 68mg, Sugar 13g, Fiber 6g

### calorie option

**350 calories:** Add an additional 2 oz chicken.

Calories 350, Carbohydrate 44g, Protein 50g, Total Fat 4g, Saturated Fat 2g, Cholesterol 89mg, Sugar 16g, Fiber 6g

## Colorful Pasta

*Serves 1.*

| | |
|---|---|
| ½ | cup cooked whole-wheat pasta |
| ⅓ | cup tomato sauce |
| ½ | cup cooked chopped spinach |
| ¼ | cup diced green bell pepper |
| ½ | cup canned white beans, rinsed and drained |
| 3 | sliced black olives |
| 1 | Tbsp Parmesan cheese |

**Combine** pasta, sauce, spinach, bell pepper, beans, and olives in a microwave-safe dish. Top with Parmesan cheese. Microwave at HIGH 1 to 2 minutes.

Calories 300, Carbohydrate 63g, Protein 21g, Total Fat 5g, Saturated Fat 1g, Cholesterol 4mg, Sugar 4g, Fiber 19g

### calorie option

**350 calories:** Add an additional 1½ Tbsp beans.

Calories 350, Carbohydrate 67g, Protein 22g, Total Fat 6g, Saturated Fat 2g, Cholesterol 4mg, Sugar 5g, Fiber 21g

## Spicy Bean Dip with Pita Triangles

*Serves 1.*

| | |
|---|---|
| 1 | cup fat-free canned refried beans (up to 115 calories) |
| ⅛ | cup light sour cream |
| ⅛ | tsp chili powder |
| ⅛ | tsp dried cumin |
| 1 | Tbsp mashed avocado |
| 1 | (6-inch) whole-wheat pita* |

**Combine** first 4 ingredients in a serving bowl. Top with avocado.

**Toast** pita and cut in triangles to use for dipping.

*About 170 calories and 4g fiber.

Calories 300, Carbohydrate 58g, Protein 15g, Total Fat 7g, Saturated Fat 3g, Cholesterol 11mg, Sugar 4g, Fiber 12g

### calorie option

**350 calories:** Add an additional ¼ cup beans.

Calories 350, Carbohydrate 63g, Protein 16g, Total Fat 9g, Saturated Fat 3g, Cholesterol 11mg, Sugar 5g, Fiber 14g

## Baby Greens with Veggie Steak Strips

*Serves 1.*

| | |
|---|---|
| 2 | cups mixed baby greens |
| ½ | cup fresh broccoli florets |
| ½ | sliced scallion |
| 4 | oz veggie steak strips |
| 1½ | tsp olive oil |
| 1 | Tbsp rice vinegar |
| 1 | Tbsp Dijon mustard |

**Combine** greens with broccoli and scallion. Heat steak strips.

**Whisk** together oil, vinegar, and mustard. Toss salad with dressing and top with steak strips.

Calories 300, Carbohydrate 15g, Protein 41g, Total Fat 12g, Saturated Fat 2g, Cholesterol 0mg, Sugar 3g, Fiber 4g

### calorie option

**350 calories:** Add an additional 1 oz veggie steak strips.

Calories 350, Carbohydrate 16g, Protein 49g, Total Fat 13g, Saturated Fat 2g, Cholesterol 0mg, Sugar 4g, Fiber 5g

# Wasabi Tuna and Spinach

*Serves 1.*

10  oz fresh loose spinach
¼   tsp wasabi powder*
1   Tbsp rice vinegar
1   Tbsp plus 1 tsp light mayonnaise
4   oz can chunk light tuna canned in
    water, drained
½   cup chopped red or yellow tomatoes

**Wash** spinach; loosely cover with a paper towel (do not dry leaves) in a microwave-safe dish. Microwave at HIGH until spinach is tender, about 1½ minutes.

Whisk together wasabi powder, vinegar, and mayonnaise. Mix into tuna. Place tuna over spinach; top with tomatoes.
*Available in the ethnic-foods sections of supermarkets.

Calories 300, Carbohydrate 20g, Protein 49g, Total Fat 8g, Saturated Fat 0.8g, Cholesterol 97mg, Sugar 3g, Fiber 7g

### calorie option

**350 calories:** Add an additional 2 oz tuna.

Calories 350, Carbohydrate 20g, Protein 62g, Total Fat 9g, Saturated Fat 0.8g, Cholesterol 127mg, Sugar 3g, Fiber 7g

# dinner recipes

## Ginger Stir-Fry

*Serves 1.*

2   tsp sesame oil

5   oz skinless, boneless chicken breast; **or** 4 oz beef tenderloin, cut in small pieces; **or** 5 oz shrimp

1½  cups Asian-style frozen vegetables

½   cup cooked brown rice

1   Tbsp rice vinegar

2   tsp fresh ginger, sliced

1   tsp reduced-sodium soy sauce

**Heat** oil in a large skillet over medium heat. Add chicken, beef, or shrimp; cook 5 to 7 minutes for chicken or beef, or 2 to 3 minutes for shrimp. Stir once or twice to cook all sides. Remove chicken, beef, or shrimp to a plate.
**Add** vegetables to pan and cook, stirring frequently, 4 to 5 minutes. Add rice, vinegar, ginger, and soy sauce. Continue to cook, stirring frequently, 2 more minutes or until heated through. Add chicken, beef, or shrimp at end to warm.

**With chicken:** Calories 400, Carbohydrate 31g, Protein 38g, Total Fat 12g, Saturated Fat 2g, Cholesterol 82mg, Sugar 2g, Fiber 5g

**With beef:** Calories 400, Carbohydrate 31g, Protein 29g, Total Fat 16g, Saturated Fat 4g, Cholesterol 61mg, Sugar 2g, Fiber 5g

**With shrimp:** Calories 400, Carbohydrate 32g, Protein 34g, Total Fat 13g, Saturated Fat 2g, Cholesterol 215mg, Sugar 2g, Fiber 5g

### calorie option

**450 calories:** Add an additional 2 oz chicken, 1½ oz beef, or 2 oz shrimp.

**With chicken:** Calories 450, Carbohydrate 31g, Protein 51g, Total Fat 13g, Saturated Fat 2g, Cholesterol 115mg, Sugar 2g, Fiber 5g

**With beef:** Calories 450, Carbohydrate 31g, Protein 39g, Total Fat 18g, Saturated Fat 4.9g, Cholesterol 83mg, Sugar 2g, Fiber 5g

**With shrimp:** Calories 450, Carbohydrate 33g, Protein 45g, Total Fat 14g, Saturated Fat 2g, Cholesterol 301mg, Sugar 2g, Fiber 5g

# Two-Mustard Chicken

*Serves 1.*

Cooking spray
1   (4-oz) skinless, boneless chicken breast
½   tsp spicy brown mustard
½   tsp Dijon mustard
2   tsp extra-virgin olive oil
¼   tsp black pepper
¼   tsp dried thyme
2   Tbsp Parmesan cheese, divided
¾   cup bulgur, cooked
½   small tomato, diced
Pinch of black pepper

**Preheat** oven to 350°F.
**Coat** a baking dish with cooking spray. Place chicken in middle of dish. Spread mustards over chicken, mixing together as you spread. Drizzle chicken with oil; sprinkle with ¼ tsp pepper, thyme, and 1 Tbsp cheese.
**Bake** at 350° for 17 to 20 minutes or until chicken is cooked through.
**Mix** bulgur with remaining 1 Tbsp cheese, tomato, and a pinch of pepper. Serve chicken on top.

Calories 400, Carbohydrate 31g, Protein 35g, Total Fat 14g, Saturated Fat 3g, Cholesterol 74mg, Sugar 3g, Fiber 8g

## calorie option

**450 calories:** Add an additional 2 oz chicken.

Calories 450, Carbohydrate 31g, Protein 48g, Total Fat 15g, Saturated Fat 4g, Cholesterol 107mg, Sugar 3g, Fiber 8g

# Sweet Pork with Apples and Broccoli

*Serves 1.*

Cooking spray
1   (5-oz) pork tenderloin
1   tsp honey
½   tsp brown sugar
1   cup fresh or frozen broccoli florets
2   Tbsp balsamic vinegar
2   Tbsp orange juice
2   tsp olive oil
1   garlic clove, minced
1   small apple, thinly sliced

**Preheat** oven to 350°F.
**Coat** a baking dish with cooking spray. Place pork in dish; top with honey and brown sugar. Arrange broccoli around pork; add vinegar, juice, oil, and garlic. Top broccoli with apple slices.
**Bake** at 350° for 30 minutes.

Calories 400, Carbohydrate 34g, Protein 35g, Total Fat 13g, Saturated Fat 2g, Cholesterol 78mg, Sugar 22g, Fiber 5g

## calorie option

**450 calories:** Add an additional 2 oz pork.

Calories 450, Carbohydrate 34g, Protein 48g, Total Fat 14g, Saturated Fat 3g, Cholesterol 109mg, Sugar 22g, Fiber 5g

# Salmon with Zucchini

*Serves 1.*

Cooking spray
1   (5-oz) salmon fillet
½   medium zucchini, thickly sliced
⅛   tsp black pepper
3   Tbsp light ranch dressing (about
     40 calories per Tbsp)

**Preheat** oven to 350°F.
**Coat** a baking dish with cooking spray.
Place fish in the middle of dish. Surround
with zucchini; sprinkle zucchini with
pepper.
**Bake** at 350° for 15 minutes. Remove
dish from oven; drizzle zucchini and fish
with dressing. Return to oven; cook 3 to
4 minutes more or until fish is opaque
and flakes easily with a fork.

Calories 400, Carbohydrate 9g, Protein 26g,
Total Fat 28g, Saturated Fat 3g, Cholesterol 86mg,
Sugar 3g, Fiber 2g

## calorie option

**450 calories:** Add an additional 1 oz salmon.

Calories 450, Carbohydrate 9g, Protein 32g,
Total Fat 31g, Saturated Fat 4g, Cholesterol 103mg,
Sugar 3g, Fiber 2g

# Orange-Glazed Salmon and Broccoli with Almonds

*Serves 1.*

Cooking spray
1   (6-oz) salmon fillet
1   Tbsp white wine or vegetable broth
1   tsp reduced-sodium soy sauce
¼   cup orange juice
1   tsp cooking sherry
¼   tsp orange zest
1   cup broccoli florets, steamed
2   Tbsp (0.64 oz) slivered almonds,
     toasted

**Preheat** oven to 400°F.
**Coat** a baking dish with cooking spray.
Place fish in dish and drizzle with white
wine or broth and soy sauce.
**Bake** at 400° for 8 to 10 minutes, or
until fish is opaque and flakes easily with
a fork.
**Coat** a small saucepan with cooking spray
and heat over medium-high heat. Add
juice, sherry, and orange zest. Cook, stirring frequently, 3 to 5 minutes or until
sauce thickens. Transfer fish and broccoli
to a serving plate; drizzle with sauce and
top with slivered almonds.

Calories 400, Carbohydrate 17g, Protein 40g,
Total Fat 18g, Saturated Fat 2g, Cholesterol 94mg,
Sugar 8g, Fiber 4g

## calorie option

**450 calories:** Add an additional 1 oz salmon
and 1 tsp almonds.

Calories 450, Carbohydrate 17g, Protein 46g,
Total Fat 21g, Saturated Fat 2.6g, Cholesterol 109mg,
Sugar 8g, Fiber 4g

## Plum Snapper with Sweet Potato Fries

*Serves 1.*

1   serving 15-Calorie Marinade (page 248)
1   (5-oz) snapper, tilapia, or halibut fillet
Cooking spray
1   (6-oz) sweet potato, cut in ½-inch-thick
    sticks
2   tsp olive oil
½   tsp paprika
½   tsp black pepper

**Preheat** oven to 350°F.

**Combine** marinade with fish in a zip-top bag. (Marinade has been calculated into the recipe. You do not need to count it as a condiment serving.) Marinate in refrigerator for 10 minutes.

**Coat** a baking dish with cooking spray. Place fries in baking dish; drizzle with oil and sprinkle with paprika and black pepper.

**Bake** at 350° for 35 minutes. Remove from oven. Place fish next to potatoes in dish; bake 10 more minutes or until fish is opaque and flakes easily with a fork.

Calories 400, Carbohydrate 41g, Protein 33g,
Total Fat 12g, Saturated Fat 2g, Cholesterol 53mg,
Sugar 12g, Fiber 6g

### calorie option

**450 calories:** Add an additional 1½ oz fish.

Calories 450, Carbohydrate 41g, Protein 42g,
Total Fat 14g, Saturated Fat 2g, Cholesterol 68mg,
Sugar 12g, Fiber 6g

## Apricot Shrimp Salad

*Serves 1.*

6   oz medium shrimp, shelled and
    deveined
1   serving 15-Calorie Marinade (page 248)
Cooking spray
1   Tbsp red wine vinegar
2   tsp olive oil
3   cups romaine lettuce
¾   cup (1½ oz) whole-wheat croutons

**Combine** shrimp with marinade in a zip-top bag. (Marinade has been calculated into the recipe. You do not need to count it as a condiment serving.) Marinate in refrigerator for at least 30 minutes. Remove shrimp from bag and discard marinade.

**Coat** a medium nonstick skillet with cooking spray. Add shrimp and cook, stirring often, 2 to 3 minutes or until shrimp turns pink.

**Toss** shrimp with vinegar and oil in a serving bowl. Place on lettuce and top with croutons.

Calories 400, Carbohydrate 26g, Protein 39g,
Total Fat 14g, Saturated Fat 2g, Cholesterol 259mg,
Sugar 6g, Fiber 5g

### calorie option

**450 calories:** Add an additional 2 oz shrimp.

Calories 450, Carbohydrate 27g, Protein 51g,
Total Fat 15g, Saturated Fat 2.4g, Cholesterol 345mg,
Sugar 6g, Fiber 5g

# chapter 12

# Success Skills Sheets & Other Essential Resources

Use the following resources as needed to follow the Complete Beck Diet for Life Program. See www.beckdietforlife.com for additional resources.

You will fill out Stages 1–5 Success Skills Sheets (pages 266–275) every night until all skills become automatic. Then you will fill out a Stage 5 Success Skills Sheet (pages 274–275) every other night, then once a week, then once a month, and then the first day of each season to keep your skills fresh. Be sure to make several copies of the Success Skills Sheet for each stage, since you may need to continue in a particular stage for several weeks. These Success Skills Sheets will keep you honest when reporting to your Diet Buddy so he/she can coach you on how to use all applicable skills the next day. Continue at a stage until you have mastered its skills for seven consecutive days.

# Sample Strength-Training Routine

Check with your doctor before starting any exercise routine.

You can do this routine at home, outdoors, in a hotel room, or in your office. It requires no equipment. Do this beginner routine twice a week to build strength. Once the exercises feel easy, either add more repetitions or a second set, or progress to a more challenging routine that incorporates dumbbells or another type of resistance.

**Push-up:** Start with your knees on the floor and your hands aligned under your shoulders. Bend your elbows as you lower your chest to the floor. Rise and repeat 8 to 10 times. Once you can easily do 10 push-ups, progress to trying a full push-up with your legs extended.

**Crunch:** Lie on your back with knees bent and hands behind your head. Exhale as you crunch up, raising your upper and middle back off the floor. Lower and repeat 10 to 15 times.

**Wall squat:** Place your back flat against a wall. Slowly walk your feet away from the wall as you bend your knees, bringing your legs to a 90° angle. Hold for 30 seconds to 2 minutes.

**Reciprocal reach:** Start with your knees on the floor and hands aligned under shoulders. Lift and extend your right arm and left leg. Hold for a count of five. Lower; then lift and extend left arm and right leg. Continue switching sides to complete 3 to 8 repetitions on each side.

**Downward facing dog:** From the reciprocal reach position, press into your hands as you lift your buttocks toward the ceiling, forming a triangle. Hold 20 seconds to 1½ minutes.

**Reverse plank:** Sit on the floor with your knees bent. Place your palms on the floor, about 6 inches behind your buttocks. Press into your hands as you raise your hips toward the ceiling, keeping your knees bent. Hold 20 seconds to 1 minute. Once you can easily hold for 1 minute in this position, progress to a full reverse plank by fully extending your legs.

**Tummy tuck:** Lie on your back with knees bent. Exhale as you pull in your tummy, as if you were trying to fit into very tight jeans. Hold for a count of five; release and repeat 10 times.

# Calorie Counts

The following Web site allows you to search an up-to-date database to find the calorie amounts of thousands of foods:

- **U.S. Department of Agriculture's Nutrient Database**
  http://www.nal.usda.gov/fnic/foodcomp/search

You can also enter the name of a food followed by the word *calories* in a search engine to find additional Web sites.

## Weight-Loss Graph

Begin to use this graph at the end of Stage 2. Create additional graphs on graph paper or in your Diet Notebook as needed.

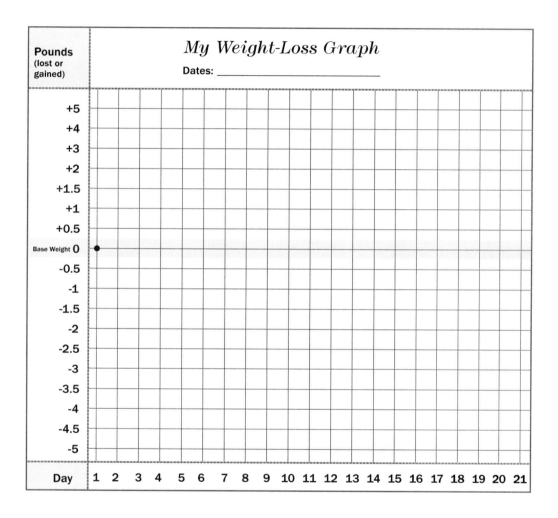

## Stage 1
## Success Skills
## Sheet

Each night, fill in every box with a symbol:

☑ If you practiced the skill fully (e.g., you ate *all* of your food sitting down, not just some of it).

☒ If you didn't practice the skill fully.

NA (not applicable) If you haven't yet learned the skill or didn't have an opportunity to practice it (e.g., maybe you were out of town and didn't have a scale or didn't need to use any Resistance Techniques).

| day____ | day____ | day____ |
|---|---|---|
| **1.** I motivated myself by reading:<br>☐ My Advantages Deck<br>☐ My Response Cards | **1.** I motivated myself by reading:<br>☐ My Advantages Deck<br>☐ My Response Cards | **1.** I motivated myself by reading:<br>☐ My Advantages Deck<br>☐ My Response Cards |
| ☐ **2.** I weighed myself just once. Weight/Change in weight: _____ | ☐ **2.** I weighed myself just once. Weight/Change in weight: _____ | ☐ **2.** I weighed myself just once. Weight/Change in weight: _____ |
| ☐ **3.** I ate everything slowly, while sitting down and enjoying every bite. | ☐ **3.** I ate everything slowly, while sitting down and enjoying every bite. | ☐ **3.** I ate everything slowly, while sitting down and enjoying every bite. |
| ☐ **4.** I gave myself credit throughout the day for every positive eating behavior. | ☐ **4.** I gave myself credit throughout the day for every positive eating behavior. | ☐ **4.** I gave myself credit throughout the day for every positive eating behavior. |
| **5.** I got moving by doing:<br>☐ Spontaneous exercise<br>☐ Planned exercise | **5.** I got moving by doing:<br>☐ Spontaneous exercise<br>☐ Planned exercise | **5.** I got moving by doing:<br>☐ Spontaneous exercise<br>☐ Planned exercise |
| ☐ **6.** I identified hunger vs. non-hunger every time I wanted to eat.<br>☐ I tolerated hunger and non-hunger without eating.<br>☐ I recognized that fullness sets in 20 minutes after a meal.<br>☐ I stopped eating when my food was gone.<br>☐ I calmed down before I ate. | ☐ **6.** I identified hunger vs. non-hunger every time I wanted to eat.<br>☐ I tolerated hunger and non-hunger without eating.<br>☐ I recognized that fullness sets in 20 minutes after a meal.<br>☐ I stopped eating when my food was gone.<br>☐ I calmed down before I ate. | ☐ **6.** I identified hunger vs. non-hunger every time I wanted to eat.<br>☐ I tolerated hunger and non-hunger without eating.<br>☐ I recognized that fullness sets in 20 minutes after a meal.<br>☐ I stopped eating when my food was gone.<br>☐ I calmed down before I ate. |
| ☐ **7.** I filled in my Food Plan Chart. | ☐ **7.** I filled in my Food Plan Chart. | ☐ **7.** I filled in my Food Plan Chart. |
| ☐ **8.** I followed my plan precisely.<br>☐ I used Resistance Techniques. | ☐ **8.** I followed my plan precisely.<br>☐ I used Resistance Techniques. | ☐ **8.** I followed my plan precisely.<br>☐ I used Resistance Techniques. |
| ☐ **9.** I got back on track.<br>☐ I filled in my Cheat Sheet. | ☐ **9.** I got back on track.<br>☐ I filled in my Cheat Sheet. | ☐ **9.** I got back on track.<br>☐ I filled in my Cheat Sheet. |
| ☐ **10.** I contacted my Diet Buddy. | ☐ **10.** I contacted my Diet Buddy. | ☐ **10.** I contacted my Diet Buddy. |

| day _____ | day _____ | day _____ | day _____ |
|---|---|---|---|
| **1.** I motivated myself by reading:<br>☐ My Advantages Deck<br>☐ My Response Cards | **1.** I motivated myself by reading:<br>☐ My Advantages Deck<br>☐ My Response Cards | **1.** I motivated myself by reading:<br>☐ My Advantages Deck<br>☐ My Response Cards | **1.** I motivated myself by reading:<br>☐ My Advantages Deck<br>☐ My Response Cards |
| ☐ **2.** I weighed myself just once. Weight/Change in weight: _____ | ☐ **2.** I weighed myself just once. Weight/Change in weight: _____ | ☐ **2.** I weighed myself just once. Weight/Change in weight: _____ | ☐ **2.** I weighed myself just once. Weight/Change in weight: _____ |
| ☐ **3.** I ate everything slowly, while sitting down and enjoying every bite. | ☐ **3.** I ate everything slowly, while sitting down and enjoying every bite. | ☐ **3.** I ate everything slowly, while sitting down and enjoying every bite. | ☐ **3.** I ate everything slowly, while sitting down and enjoying every bite. |
| ☐ **4.** I gave myself credit throughout the day for every positive eating behavior. | ☐ **4.** I gave myself credit throughout the day for every positive eating behavior. | ☐ **4.** I gave myself credit throughout the day for every positive eating behavior. | ☐ **4.** I gave myself credit throughout the day for every positive eating behavior. |
| **5.** I got moving by doing:<br>☐ Spontaneous exercise<br>☐ Planned exercise | **5.** I got moving by doing:<br>☐ Spontaneous exercise<br>☐ Planned exercise | **5.** I got moving by doing:<br>☐ Spontaneous exercise<br>☐ Planned exercise | **5.** I got moving by doing:<br>☐ Spontaneous exercise<br>☐ Planned exercise |
| ☐ **6.** I identified hunger vs. non-hunger every time I wanted to eat.<br>☐ I tolerated hunger and non-hunger without eating.<br>☐ I recognized that fullness sets in 20 minutes after a meal.<br>☐ I stopped eating when my food was gone.<br>☐ I calmed down before I ate. | ☐ **6.** I identified hunger vs. non-hunger every time I wanted to eat.<br>☐ I tolerated hunger and non-hunger without eating.<br>☐ I recognized that fullness sets in 20 minutes after a meal.<br>☐ I stopped eating when my food was gone.<br>☐ I calmed down before I ate. | ☐ **6.** I identified hunger vs. non-hunger every time I wanted to eat.<br>☐ I tolerated hunger and non-hunger without eating.<br>☐ I recognized that fullness sets in 20 minutes after a meal.<br>☐ I stopped eating when my food was gone.<br>☐ I calmed down before I ate. | ☐ **6.** I identified hunger vs. non-hunger every time I wanted to eat.<br>☐ I tolerated hunger and non-hunger without eating.<br>☐ I recognized that fullness sets in 20 minutes after a meal.<br>☐ I stopped eating when my food was gone.<br>☐ I calmed down before I ate. |
| ☐ **7.** I filled in my Food Plan Chart. | ☐ **7.** I filled in my Food Plan Chart. | ☐ **7.** I filled in my Food Plan Chart. | ☐ **7.** I filled in my Food Plan Chart. |
| ☐ **8.** I followed my plan precisely.<br>☐ I used Resistance Techniques. | ☐ **8.** I followed my plan precisely.<br>☐ I used Resistance Techniques. | ☐ **8.** I followed my plan precisely.<br>☐ I used Resistance Techniques. | ☐ **8.** I followed my plan precisely.<br>☐ I used Resistance Techniques. |
| ☐ **9.** I got back on track.<br>☐ I filled in my Cheat Sheet. | ☐ **9.** I got back on track.<br>☐ I filled in my Cheat Sheet. | ☐ **9.** I got back on track.<br>☐ I filled in my Cheat Sheet. | ☐ **9.** I got back on track.<br>☐ I filled in my Cheat Sheet. |
| ☐ **10.** I contacted my Diet Buddy. | ☐ **10.** I contacted my Diet Buddy. | ☐ **10.** I contacted my Diet Buddy. | ☐ **10.** I contacted my Diet Buddy. |

## Stage 2 Success Skills Sheet

Each night, fill in every box with a symbol:

☑ If you practiced the skill fully (e.g., you ate *all* of your food sitting down, not just some of it).

☒ If you didn't practice the skill fully.

NA (not applicable) If you haven't yet learned the skill or didn't have an opportunity to practice it (e.g., maybe you were out of town and didn't have a scale or didn't need to use any Resistance Techniques).

---

### day_____

**1.** I motivated myself by reading:
- ☐ My Advantages Deck
- ☐ My Response Cards

**2.** I weighed myself just once. Weight/Change in weight: _____

**3.** I ate everything slowly, while sitting down and enjoying every bite.

**4.** I gave myself credit throughout the day for every positive eating behavior.

**5.** I got moving by doing:
- ☐ Spontaneous exercise
- ☐ Planned exercise

**6.** ☐ I identified hunger vs. non-hunger every time I wanted to eat.
- ☐ I tolerated hunger and non-hunger without eating.
- ☐ I recognized that fullness sets in 20 minutes after a meal.
- ☐ I stopped eating when my food was gone.
- ☐ I calmed down before I ate.

**7.** ☐ I filled in my Food Plan Chart.

**8.** ☐ I followed my plan precisely.
- ☐ I measured every portion.
- ☐ I used Resistance Techniques.
- ☐ I recorded all unplanned eating.

**9.** ☐ I got back on track.
- ☐ I filled in my Cheat Sheet.

**10.** ☐ I contacted my Diet Buddy.

---

### day_____

**1.** I motivated myself by reading:
- ☐ My Advantages Deck
- ☐ My Response Cards

**2.** I weighed myself just once. Weight/Change in weight: _____

**3.** I ate everything slowly, while sitting down and enjoying every bite.

**4.** I gave myself credit throughout the day for every positive eating behavior.

**5.** I got moving by doing:
- ☐ Spontaneous exercise
- ☐ Planned exercise

**6.** ☐ I identified hunger vs. non-hunger every time I wanted to eat.
- ☐ I tolerated hunger and non-hunger without eating.
- ☐ I recognized that fullness sets in 20 minutes after a meal.
- ☐ I stopped eating when my food was gone.
- ☐ I calmed down before I ate.

**7.** ☐ I filled in my Food Plan Chart.

**8.** ☐ I followed my plan precisely.
- ☐ I measured every portion.
- ☐ I used Resistance Techniques.
- ☐ I recorded all unplanned eating.

**9.** ☐ I got back on track.
- ☐ I filled in my Cheat Sheet.

**10.** ☐ I contacted my Diet Buddy.

---

### day_____

**1.** I motivated myself by reading:
- ☐ My Advantages Deck
- ☐ My Response Cards

**2.** I weighed myself just once. Weight/Change in weight: _____

**3.** I ate everything slowly, while sitting down and enjoying every bite.

**4.** I gave myself credit throughout the day for every positive eating behavior.

**5.** I got moving by doing:
- ☐ Spontaneous exercise
- ☐ Planned exercise

**6.** ☐ I identified hunger vs. non-hunger every time I wanted to eat.
- ☐ I tolerated hunger and non-hunger without eating.
- ☐ I recognized that fullness sets in 20 minutes after a meal.
- ☐ I stopped eating when my food was gone.
- ☐ I calmed down before I ate.

**7.** ☐ I filled in my Food Plan Chart.

**8.** ☐ I followed my plan precisely.
- ☐ I measured every portion.
- ☐ I used Resistance Techniques.
- ☐ I recorded all unplanned eating.

**9.** ☐ I got back on track.
- ☐ I filled in my Cheat Sheet.

**10.** ☐ I contacted my Diet Buddy.

## day____

1. I motivated myself by reading:
- ☐ My Advantages Deck
- ☐ My Response Cards

☐ **2.** I weighed myself just once. Weight/Change in weight: ____________

☐ **3.** I ate everything slowly, while sitting down and enjoying every bite.

☐ **4.** I gave myself credit throughout the day for every positive eating behavior.

**5.** I got moving by doing:
- ☐ Spontaneous exercise
- ☐ Planned exercise

☐ **6.** I identified hunger vs. non-hunger every time I wanted to eat.
- ☐ I tolerated hunger and non-hunger without eating.
- ☐ I recognized that fullness sets in 20 minutes after a meal.
- ☐ I stopped eating when my food was gone.
- ☐ I calmed down before I ate.

☐ **7.** I filled in my Food Plan Chart.

☐ **8.** I followed my plan precisely.
- ☐ I measured every portion.
- ☐ I used Resistance Techniques.
- ☐ I recorded all unplanned eating.

☐ **9.** I got back on track.
- ☐ I filled in my Cheat Sheet.

☐ **10.** I contacted my Diet Buddy.


## day____

1. I motivated myself by reading:
- ☐ My Advantages Deck
- ☐ My Response Cards

☐ **2.** I weighed myself just once. Weight/Change in weight: ____________

☐ **3.** I ate everything slowly, while sitting down and enjoying every bite.

☐ **4.** I gave myself credit throughout the day for every positive eating behavior.

**5.** I got moving by doing:
- ☐ Spontaneous exercise
- ☐ Planned exercise

☐ **6.** I identified hunger vs. non-hunger every time I wanted to eat.
- ☐ I tolerated hunger and non-hunger without eating.
- ☐ I recognized that fullness sets in 20 minutes after a meal.
- ☐ I stopped eating when my food was gone.
- ☐ I calmed down before I ate.

☐ **7.** I filled in my Food Plan Chart.

☐ **8.** I followed my plan precisely.
- ☐ I measured every portion.
- ☐ I used Resistance Techniques.
- ☐ I recorded all unplanned eating.

☐ **9.** I got back on track.
- ☐ I filled in my Cheat Sheet.

☐ **10.** I contacted my Diet Buddy.



## day____

1. I motivated myself by reading:
- ☐ My Advantages Deck
- ☐ My Response Cards

☐ **2.** I weighed myself just once. Weight/Change in weight: ____________

☐ **3.** I ate everything slowly, while sitting down and enjoying every bite.

☐ **4.** I gave myself credit throughout the day for every positive eating behavior.

**5.** I got moving by doing:
- ☐ Spontaneous exercise
- ☐ Planned exercise

☐ **6.** I identified hunger vs. non-hunger every time I wanted to eat.
- ☐ I tolerated hunger and non-hunger without eating.
- ☐ I recognized that fullness sets in 20 minutes after a meal.
- ☐ I stopped eating when my food was gone.
- ☐ I calmed down before I ate.

☐ **7.** I filled in my Food Plan Chart.

☐ **8.** I followed my plan precisely.
- ☐ I measured every portion.
- ☐ I used Resistance Techniques.
- ☐ I recorded all unplanned eating.

☐ **9.** I got back on track.
- ☐ I filled in my Cheat Sheet.

☐ **10.** I contacted my Diet Buddy.



## day____

1. I motivated myself by reading:
- ☐ My Advantages Deck
- ☐ My Response Cards

☐ **2.** I weighed myself just once. Weight/Change in weight: ____________

☐ **3.** I ate everything slowly, while sitting down and enjoying every bite.

☐ **4.** I gave myself credit throughout the day for every positive eating behavior.

**5.** I got moving by doing:
- ☐ Spontaneous exercise
- ☐ Planned exercise

☐ **6.** I identified hunger vs. non-hunger every time I wanted to eat.
- ☐ I tolerated hunger and non-hunger without eating.
- ☐ I recognized that fullness sets in 20 minutes after a meal.
- ☐ I stopped eating when my food was gone.
- ☐ I calmed down before I ate.

☐ **7.** I filled in my Food Plan Chart.

☐ **8.** I followed my plan precisely.
- ☐ I measured every portion.
- ☐ I used Resistance Techniques.
- ☐ I recorded all unplanned eating.

☐ **9.** I got back on track.
- ☐ I filled in my Cheat Sheet.

☐ **10.** I contacted my Diet Buddy.

## Stage 3 Success Skills Sheet

**E**ach night, fill in every box with a symbol:

☑ If you practiced the skill fully (e.g., you ate *all* of your food sitting down, not just some of it).

☒ If you didn't practice the skill fully.

NA (not applicable) If you haven't yet learned the skill or didn't have an opportunity to practice it (e.g., maybe you were out of town and didn't have a scale or didn't need to use any Resistance Techniques).

| day_____ | day_____ | day_____ |
|---|---|---|
| **1.** I motivated myself by reading:<br>☐ My Advantages Deck<br>☐ My Response Cards | **1.** I motivated myself by reading:<br>☐ My Advantages Deck<br>☐ My Response Cards | **1.** I motivated myself by reading:<br>☐ My Advantages Deck<br>☐ My Response Cards |
| ☐ **2.** I weighed myself just once. Weight/Change in weight: _____ | ☐ **2.** I weighed myself just once. Weight/Change in weight: _____ | ☐ **2.** I weighed myself just once. Weight/Change in weight: _____ |
| ☐ **3.** I ate everything slowly, while sitting down and enjoying every bite. | ☐ **3.** I ate everything slowly, while sitting down and enjoying every bite. | ☐ **3.** I ate everything slowly, while sitting down and enjoying every bite. |
| ☐ **4.** I gave myself credit throughout the day for every positive eating behavior. | ☐ **4.** I gave myself credit throughout the day for every positive eating behavior. | ☐ **4.** I gave myself credit throughout the day for every positive eating behavior. |
| **5.** I got moving by doing:<br>☐ Spontaneous exercise<br>☐ Planned exercise | **5.** I got moving by doing:<br>☐ Spontaneous exercise<br>☐ Planned exercise | **5.** I got moving by doing:<br>☐ Spontaneous exercise<br>☐ Planned exercise |
| ☐ **6.** I identified hunger vs. non-hunger every time I wanted to eat.<br>☐ I tolerated hunger and non-hunger without eating.<br>☐ I recognized that fullness sets in 20 minutes after a meal.<br>☐ I stopped eating when my food was gone.<br>☐ I calmed down before I ate. | ☐ **6.** I identified hunger vs. non-hunger every time I wanted to eat.<br>☐ I tolerated hunger and non-hunger without eating.<br>☐ I recognized that fullness sets in 20 minutes after a meal.<br>☐ I stopped eating when my food was gone.<br>☐ I calmed down before I ate. | ☐ **6.** I identified hunger vs. non-hunger every time I wanted to eat.<br>☐ I tolerated hunger and non-hunger without eating.<br>☐ I recognized that fullness sets in 20 minutes after a meal.<br>☐ I stopped eating when my food was gone.<br>☐ I calmed down before I ate. |
| ☐ **7.** I filled in my Food Plan Chart. | ☐ **7.** I filled in my Food Plan Chart. | ☐ **7.** I filled in my Food Plan Chart. |
| ☐ **8.** I followed my plan precisely.<br>☐ I measured every portion.<br>☐ I followed my Challenging Situations Plan.<br>☐ I used Resistance Techniques.<br>☐ I recorded all unplanned eating. | ☐ **8.** I followed my plan precisely.<br>☐ I measured every portion.<br>☐ I followed my Challenging Situations Plan.<br>☐ I used Resistance Techniques.<br>☐ I recorded all unplanned eating. | ☐ **8.** I followed my plan precisely.<br>☐ I measured every portion.<br>☐ I followed my Challenging Situations Plan.<br>☐ I used Resistance Techniques.<br>☐ I recorded all unplanned eating. |
| ☐ **9.** I got back on track.<br>☐ I filled in my Cheat Sheet. | ☐ **9.** I got back on track.<br>☐ I filled in my Cheat Sheet. | ☐ **9.** I got back on track.<br>☐ I filled in my Cheat Sheet. |
| ☐ **10.** I contacted my Diet Buddy. | ☐ **10.** I contacted my Diet Buddy. | ☐ **10.** I contacted my Diet Buddy. |

| day___ | day___ | day___ | day___ |
|---|---|---|---|
| **1.** I motivated myself by reading:<br>☐ My Advantages Deck<br>☐ My Response Cards | **1.** I motivated myself by reading:<br>☐ My Advantages Deck<br>☐ My Response Cards | **1.** I motivated myself by reading:<br>☐ My Advantages Deck<br>☐ My Response Cards | **1.** I motivated myself by reading:<br>☐ My Advantages Deck<br>☐ My Response Cards |
| ☐ **2.** I weighed myself just once. Weight/Change in weight: _____ | ☐ **2.** I weighed myself just once. Weight/Change in weight: _____ | ☐ **2.** I weighed myself just once. Weight/Change in weight: _____ | ☐ **2.** I weighed myself just once. Weight/Change in weight: _____ |
| ☐ **3.** I ate everything slowly, while sitting down and enjoying every bite. | ☐ **3.** I ate everything slowly, while sitting down and enjoying every bite. | ☐ **3.** I ate everything slowly, while sitting down and enjoying every bite. | ☐ **3.** I ate everything slowly, while sitting down and enjoying every bite. |
| ☐ **4.** I gave myself credit throughout the day for every positive eating behavior. | ☐ **4.** I gave myself credit throughout the day for every positive eating behavior. | ☐ **4.** I gave myself credit throughout the day for every positive eating behavior. | ☐ **4.** I gave myself credit throughout the day for every positive eating behavior. |
| **5.** I got moving by doing:<br>☐ Spontaneous exercise<br>☐ Planned exercise | **5.** I got moving by doing:<br>☐ Spontaneous exercise<br>☐ Planned exercise | **5.** I got moving by doing:<br>☐ Spontaneous exercise<br>☐ Planned exercise | **5.** I got moving by doing:<br>☐ Spontaneous exercise<br>☐ Planned exercise |
| ☐ **6.** I identified hunger vs. non-hunger every time I wanted to eat.<br>☐ I tolerated hunger and non-hunger without eating.<br>☐ I recognized that fullness sets in 20 minutes after a meal.<br>☐ I stopped eating when my food was gone.<br>☐ I calmed down before I ate. | ☐ **6.** I identified hunger vs. non-hunger every time I wanted to eat.<br>☐ I tolerated hunger and non-hunger without eating.<br>☐ I recognized that fullness sets in 20 minutes after a meal.<br>☐ I stopped eating when my food was gone.<br>☐ I calmed down before I ate. | ☐ **6.** I identified hunger vs. non-hunger every time I wanted to eat.<br>☐ I tolerated hunger and non-hunger without eating.<br>☐ I recognized that fullness sets in 20 minutes after a meal.<br>☐ I stopped eating when my food was gone.<br>☐ I calmed down before I ate. | ☐ **6.** I identified hunger vs. non-hunger every time I wanted to eat.<br>☐ I tolerated hunger and non-hunger without eating.<br>☐ I recognized that fullness sets in 20 minutes after a meal.<br>☐ I stopped eating when my food was gone.<br>☐ I calmed down before I ate. |
| ☐ **7.** I filled in my Food Plan Chart. | ☐ **7.** I filled in my Food Plan Chart. | ☐ **7.** I filled in my Food Plan Chart. | ☐ **7.** I filled in my Food Plan Chart. |
| ☐ **8.** I followed my plan precisely.<br>☐ I measured every portion.<br>☐ I followed my Challenging Situations Plan.<br>☐ I used Resistance Techniques.<br>☐ I recorded all unplanned eating. | ☐ **8.** I followed my plan precisely.<br>☐ I measured every portion.<br>☐ I followed my Challenging Situations Plan.<br>☐ I used Resistance Techniques.<br>☐ I recorded all unplanned eating. | ☐ **8.** I followed my plan precisely.<br>☐ I measured every portion.<br>☐ I followed my Challenging Situations Plan.<br>☐ I used Resistance Techniques.<br>☐ I recorded all unplanned eating. | ☐ **8.** I followed my plan precisely.<br>☐ I measured every portion.<br>☐ I followed my Challenging Situations Plan.<br>☐ I used Resistance Techniques.<br>☐ I recorded all unplanned eating. |
| ☐ **9.** I got back on track.<br>☐ I filled in my Cheat Sheet. | ☐ **9.** I got back on track.<br>☐ I filled in my Cheat Sheet. | ☐ **9.** I got back on track.<br>☐ I filled in my Cheat Sheet. | ☐ **9.** I got back on track.<br>☐ I filled in my Cheat Sheet. |
| ☐ **10.** I contacted my Diet Buddy. | ☐ **10.** I contacted my Diet Buddy. | ☐ **10.** I contacted my Diet Buddy. | ☐ **10.** I contacted my Diet Buddy. |

## Stage 4
## Success Skills
## Sheet

**E**ach night, fill in every box with a symbol:

☑ If you practiced the skill fully (e.g., you ate *all* of your food sitting down, not just some of it).

☒ If you didn't practice the skill fully.

NA (not applicable) If you haven't yet learned the skill or didn't have an opportunity to practice it (e.g., maybe you were out of town and didn't have a scale or didn't need to use any Resistance Techniques).

| day_____ | day_____ | day_____ |
|---|---|---|
| **1.** I motivated myself by reading: <br>☐ My Advantages Deck <br>☐ My Response Cards | **1.** I motivated myself by reading: <br>☐ My Advantages Deck <br>☐ My Response Cards | **1.** I motivated myself by reading: <br>☐ My Advantages Deck <br>☐ My Response Cards |
| ☐ **2.** I weighed myself just once. Weight/Change in weight: _____ | ☐ **2.** I weighed myself just once. Weight/Change in weight: _____ | ☐ **2.** I weighed myself just once. Weight/Change in weight: _____ |
| ☐ **3.** I ate everything slowly, while sitting down and enjoying every bite. | ☐ **3.** I ate everything slowly, while sitting down and enjoying every bite. | ☐ **3.** I ate everything slowly, while sitting down and enjoying every bite. |
| ☐ **4.** I gave myself credit for every positive eating behavior. | ☐ **4.** I gave myself credit for every positive eating behavior. | ☐ **4.** I gave myself credit for every positive eating behavior. |
| **5.** I got moving by doing: <br>☐ Spontaneous exercise <br>☐ Planned exercise | **5.** I got moving by doing: <br>☐ Spontaneous exercise <br>☐ Planned exercise | **5.** I got moving by doing: <br>☐ Spontaneous exercise <br>☐ Planned exercise |
| ☐ **6.** I identified hunger vs. non-hunger every time I wanted to eat. <br>☐ I tolerated hunger and non-hunger without eating. <br>☐ I recognized that fullness sets in 20 minutes after a meal. <br>☐ I stopped eating when my food was gone. <br>☐ I calmed down before I ate. | ☐ **6.** I identified hunger vs. non-hunger every time I wanted to eat. <br>☐ I tolerated hunger and non-hunger without eating. <br>☐ I recognized that fullness sets in 20 minutes after a meal. <br>☐ I stopped eating when my food was gone. <br>☐ I calmed down before I ate. | ☐ **6.** I identified hunger vs. non-hunger every time I wanted to eat. <br>☐ I tolerated hunger and non-hunger without eating. <br>☐ I recognized that fullness sets in 20 minutes after a meal. <br>☐ I stopped eating when my food was gone. <br>☐ I calmed down before I ate. |
| ☐ **7.** I filled in my Food Plan Chart **OR** made a mental plan. | ☐ **7.** I filled in my Food Plan Chart **OR** made a mental plan. | ☐ **7.** I filled in my Food Plan Chart **OR** made a mental plan. |
| ☐ **8.** I followed my plan precisely **OR** I made legitimate changes. <br>☐ I measured every portion. <br>☐ I followed my Challenging Situations Plan. <br>☐ I used Resistance Techniques. <br>☐ I recorded all unplanned eating. | ☐ **8.** I followed my plan precisely **OR** I made legitimate changes. <br>☐ I measured every portion. <br>☐ I followed my Challenging Situations Plan. <br>☐ I used Resistance Techniques. <br>☐ I recorded all unplanned eating. | ☐ **8.** I followed my plan precisely **OR** I made legitimate changes. <br>☐ I measured every portion. <br>☐ I followed my Challenging Situations Plan. <br>☐ I used Resistance Techniques. <br>☐ I recorded all unplanned eating. |
| ☐ **9.** I got back on track. <br>☐ I filled in my Cheat Sheet. | ☐ **9.** I got back on track. <br>☐ I filled in my Cheat Sheet. | ☐ **9.** I got back on track. <br>☐ I filled in my Cheat Sheet. |
| ☐ **10.** I contacted my Diet Buddy. | ☐ **10.** I contacted my Diet Buddy. | ☐ **10.** I contacted my Diet Buddy. |

# day____

**1.** I motivated myself by reading:
- [ ] My Advantages Deck
- [ ] My Response Cards

- [ ] **2.** I weighed myself just once. Weight/Change in weight: _____

- [ ] **3.** I ate everything slowly, while sitting down and enjoying every bite.

- [ ] **4.** I gave myself credit for every positive eating behavior.

**5.** I got moving by doing:
- [ ] Spontaneous exercise
- [ ] Planned exercise

- [ ] **6.** I identified hunger vs. non-hunger every time I wanted to eat.
- [ ] I tolerated hunger and non-hunger without eating.
- [ ] I recognized that fullness sets in 20 minutes after a meal.
- [ ] I stopped eating when my food was gone.
- [ ] I calmed down before I ate.

- [ ] **7.** I filled in my Food Plan Chart **OR** made a mental plan.

- [ ] **8.** I followed my plan precisely **OR** I made legitimate changes.
- [ ] I measured every portion.
- [ ] I followed my Challenging Situations Plan.
- [ ] I used Resistance Techniques.
- [ ] I recorded all unplanned eating.

- [ ] **9.** I got back on track.
- [ ] I filled in my Cheat Sheet.

- [ ] **10.** I contacted my Diet Buddy.

# day____

**1.** I motivated myself by reading:
- [ ] My Advantages Deck
- [ ] My Response Cards

- [ ] **2.** I weighed myself just once. Weight/Change in weight: _____

- [ ] **3.** I ate everything slowly, while sitting down and enjoying every bite.

- [ ] **4.** I gave myself credit for every positive eating behavior.

**5.** I got moving by doing:
- [ ] Spontaneous exercise
- [ ] Planned exercise

- [ ] **6.** I identified hunger vs. non-hunger every time I wanted to eat.
- [ ] I tolerated hunger and non-hunger without eating.
- [ ] I recognized that fullness sets in 20 minutes after a meal.
- [ ] I stopped eating when my food was gone.
- [ ] I calmed down before I ate.

- [ ] **7.** I filled in my Food Plan Chart **OR** made a mental plan.

- [ ] **8.** I followed my plan precisely **OR** I made legitimate changes.
- [ ] I measured every portion.
- [ ] I followed my Challenging Situations Plan.
- [ ] I used Resistance Techniques.
- [ ] I recorded all unplanned eating.

- [ ] **9.** I got back on track.
- [ ] I filled in my Cheat Sheet.

- [ ] **10.** I contacted my Diet Buddy.

# day____

**1.** I motivated myself by reading:
- [ ] My Advantages Deck
- [ ] My Response Cards

- [ ] **2.** I weighed myself just once. Weight/Change in weight: _____

- [ ] **3.** I ate everything slowly, while sitting down and enjoying every bite.

- [ ] **4.** I gave myself credit for every positive eating behavior.

**5.** I got moving by doing:
- [ ] Spontaneous exercise
- [ ] Planned exercise

- [ ] **6.** I identified hunger vs. non-hunger every time I wanted to eat.
- [ ] I tolerated hunger and non-hunger without eating.
- [ ] I recognized that fullness sets in 20 minutes after a meal.
- [ ] I stopped eating when my food was gone.
- [ ] I calmed down before I ate.

- [ ] **7.** I filled in my Food Plan Chart **OR** made a mental plan.

- [ ] **8.** I followed my plan precisely **OR** I made legitimate changes.
- [ ] I measured every portion.
- [ ] I followed my Challenging Situations Plan.
- [ ] I used Resistance Techniques.
- [ ] I recorded all unplanned eating.

- [ ] **9.** I got back on track.
- [ ] I filled in my Cheat Sheet.

- [ ] **10.** I contacted my Diet Buddy.

# day____

**1.** I motivated myself by reading:
- [ ] My Advantages Deck
- [ ] My Response Cards

- [ ] **2.** I weighed myself just once. Weight/Change in weight: _____

- [ ] **3.** I ate everything slowly, while sitting down and enjoying every bite.

- [ ] **4.** I gave myself credit for every positive eating behavior.

**5.** I got moving by doing:
- [ ] Spontaneous exercise
- [ ] Planned exercise

- [ ] **6.** I identified hunger vs. non-hunger every time I wanted to eat.
- [ ] I tolerated hunger and non-hunger without eating.
- [ ] I recognized that fullness sets in 20 minutes after a meal.
- [ ] I stopped eating when my food was gone.
- [ ] I calmed down before I ate.

- [ ] **7.** I filled in my Food Plan Chart **OR** made a mental plan.

- [ ] **8.** I followed my plan precisely **OR** I made legitimate changes.
- [ ] I measured every portion.
- [ ] I followed my Challenging Situations Plan.
- [ ] I used Resistance Techniques.
- [ ] I recorded all unplanned eating.

- [ ] **9.** I got back on track.
- [ ] I filled in my Cheat Sheet.

- [ ] **10.** I contacted my Diet Buddy.

## Stage 5
## Success Skills
## Sheet

Each night, fill in every box with a symbol:

☑ If you practiced the skill fully (e.g., you ate *all* of your food sitting down, not just some of it).

☒ If you didn't practice the skill fully.

NA (not applicable) If you haven't yet learned the skill or didn't have an opportunity to practice it (e.g., maybe you were out of town and didn't have a scale or didn't need to use any Resistance Techniques).

### day_____

**1.** I motivated myself by:
☐ Reading my Advantages Deck and my Response Cards
☐ Practicing my Daily Motivation Plan

**2.** I weighed myself just once. Weight/Change in weight: _____

**3.** I ate everything slowly, while sitting down and enjoying every bite.

**4.** I gave myself credit for every positive eating behavior.

**5.** I got moving by doing:
☐ Spontaneous exercise
☐ Planned exercise

**6.** I identified hunger vs. non-hunger every time I wanted to eat.
☐ I tolerated hunger and non-hunger without eating.
☐ I recognized fullness sets in after 20 minutes.
☐ I stopped eating when my food was gone.
☐ I calmed down before I ate.

**7.** I filled in my Food Plan Chart **OR** made a mental plan.

**8.** I followed my plan precisely **OR** I made legitimate changes.
☐ I measured every portion.
☐ I followed my Challenging Situations Plan.
☐ I used Resistance Techniques.
☐ I recorded all unplanned eating.

**9.** I got back on track.
☐ I filled in my Cheat Sheet.

**10.** I contacted my Diet Buddy.

### day_____

**1.** I motivated myself by:
☐ Reading my Advantages Deck and my Response Cards
☐ Practicing my Daily Motivation Plan

**2.** I weighed myself just once. Weight/Change in weight: _____

**3.** I ate everything slowly, while sitting down and enjoying every bite.

**4.** I gave myself credit for every positive eating behavior.

**5.** I got moving by doing:
☐ Spontaneous exercise
☐ Planned exercise

**6.** I identified hunger vs. non-hunger every time I wanted to eat.
☐ I tolerated hunger and non-hunger without eating.
☐ I recognized fullness sets in after 20 minutes.
☐ I stopped eating when my food was gone.
☐ I calmed down before I ate.

**7.** I filled in my Food Plan Chart **OR** made a mental plan.

**8.** I followed my plan precisely **OR** I made legitimate changes.
☐ I measured every portion.
☐ I followed my Challenging Situations Plan.
☐ I used Resistance Techniques.
☐ I recorded all unplanned eating.

**9.** I got back on track.
☐ I filled in my Cheat Sheet.

**10.** I contacted my Diet Buddy.

### day_____

**1.** I motivated myself by:
☐ Reading my Advantages Deck and my Response Cards
☐ Practicing my Daily Motivation Plan

**2.** I weighed myself just once. Weight/Change in weight: _____

**3.** I ate everything slowly, while sitting down and enjoying every bite.

**4.** I gave myself credit for every positive eating behavior.

**5.** I got moving by doing:
☐ Spontaneous exercise
☐ Planned exercise

**6.** I identified hunger vs. non-hunger every time I wanted to eat.
☐ I tolerated hunger and non-hunger without eating.
☐ I recognized fullness sets in after 20 minutes.
☐ I stopped eating when my food was gone.
☐ I calmed down before I ate.

**7.** I filled in my Food Plan Chart **OR** made a mental plan.

**8.** I followed my plan precisely **OR** I made legitimate changes.
☐ I measured every portion.
☐ I followed my Challenging Situations Plan.
☐ I used Resistance Techniques.
☐ I recorded all unplanned eating.

**9.** I got back on track.
☐ I filled in my Cheat Sheet.

**10.** I contacted my Diet Buddy.

| day _____ | day _____ | day _____ | day _____ |
|---|---|---|---|
| **1.** I motivated myself by:<br>☐ Reading my **Advantages Deck** and my **Response Cards**<br>☐ Practicing my **Daily Motivation Plan** | **1.** I motivated myself by:<br>☐ Reading my **Advantages Deck** and my **Response Cards**<br>☐ Practicing my **Daily Motivation Plan** | **1.** I motivated myself by:<br>☐ Reading my **Advantages Deck** and my **Response Cards**<br>☐ Practicing my **Daily Motivation Plan** | **1.** I motivated myself by:<br>☐ Reading my **Advantages Deck** and my **Response Cards**<br>☐ Practicing my **Daily Motivation Plan** |
| ☐ **2.** I weighed myself just once. **Weight/Change** in weight: _____ | ☐ **2.** I weighed myself just once. **Weight/Change** in weight: _____ | ☐ **2.** I weighed myself just once. **Weight/Change** in weight: _____ | ☐ **2.** I weighed myself just once. **Weight/Change** in weight: _____ |
| ☐ **3.** I ate everything slowly, while sitting down and enjoying every bite. | ☐ **3.** I ate everything slowly, while sitting down and enjoying every bite. | ☐ **3.** I ate everything slowly, while sitting down and enjoying every bite. | ☐ **3.** I ate everything slowly, while sitting down and enjoying every bite. |
| ☐ **4.** I gave myself credit for every positive eating behavior. | ☐ **4.** I gave myself credit for every positive eating behavior. | ☐ **4.** I gave myself credit for every positive eating behavior. | ☐ **4.** I gave myself credit for every positive eating behavior. |
| **5.** I got moving by doing:<br>☐ Spontaneous exercise<br>☐ Planned exercise | **5.** I got moving by doing:<br>☐ Spontaneous exercise<br>☐ Planned exercise | **5.** I got moving by doing:<br>☐ Spontaneous exercise<br>☐ Planned exercise | **5.** I got moving by doing:<br>☐ Spontaneous exercise<br>☐ Planned exercise |
| ☐ **6.** I identified hunger vs. non-hunger every time I wanted to eat.<br>☐ I tolerated hunger and non-hunger without eating.<br>☐ I recognized fullness sets in after 20 minutes.<br>☐ I stopped eating when my food was gone.<br>☐ I calmed down before I ate. | ☐ **6.** I identified hunger vs. non-hunger every time I wanted to eat.<br>☐ I tolerated hunger and non-hunger without eating.<br>☐ I recognized fullness sets in after 20 minutes.<br>☐ I stopped eating when my food was gone.<br>☐ I calmed down before I ate. | ☐ **6.** I identified hunger vs. non-hunger every time I wanted to eat.<br>☐ I tolerated hunger and non-hunger without eating.<br>☐ I recognized fullness sets in after 20 minutes.<br>☐ I stopped eating when my food was gone.<br>☐ I calmed down before I ate. | ☐ **6.** I identified hunger vs. non-hunger every time I wanted to eat.<br>☐ I tolerated hunger and non-hunger without eating.<br>☐ I recognized fullness sets in after 20 minutes.<br>☐ I stopped eating when my food was gone.<br>☐ I calmed down before I ate. |
| ☐ **7.** I filled in my Food Plan Chart **OR** made a mental plan. | ☐ **7.** I filled in my Food Plan Chart **OR** made a mental plan. | ☐ **7.** I filled in my Food Plan Chart **OR** made a mental plan. | ☐ **7.** I filled in my Food Plan Chart **OR** made a mental plan. |
| ☐ **8.** I followed my plan precisely **OR** I made legitimate changes.<br>☐ I measured every portion.<br>☐ I followed my Challenging Situations Plan.<br>☐ I used Resistance Techniques.<br>☐ I recorded all unplanned eating. | ☐ **8.** I followed my plan precisely **OR** I made legitimate changes.<br>☐ I measured every portion.<br>☐ I followed my Challenging Situations Plan.<br>☐ I used Resistance Techniques.<br>☐ I recorded all unplanned eating. | ☐ **8.** I followed my plan precisely **OR** I made legitimate changes.<br>☐ I measured every portion.<br>☐ I followed my Challenging Situations Plan.<br>☐ I used Resistance Techniques.<br>☐ I recorded all unplanned eating. | ☐ **8.** I followed my plan precisely **OR** I made legitimate changes.<br>☐ I measured every portion.<br>☐ I followed my Challenging Situations Plan.<br>☐ I used Resistance Techniques.<br>☐ I recorded all unplanned eating. |
| ☐ **9.** I got back on track.<br>☐ I filled in my Cheat Sheet. | ☐ **9.** I got back on track.<br>☐ I filled in my Cheat Sheet. | ☐ **9.** I got back on track.<br>☐ I filled in my Cheat Sheet. | ☐ **9.** I got back on track.<br>☐ I filled in my Cheat Sheet. |
| ☐ **10.** I contacted my Diet Buddy. | ☐ **10.** I contacted my Diet Buddy. | ☐ **10.** I contacted my Diet Buddy. | ☐ **10.** I contacted my Diet Buddy. |

# Selected Bibliography

## Chapter 1: Begin a New Way of Life

Claudino, A.M.; de Oliveira, I.R.; Appolinaro, J.C.; Cordas, T.A.; Duchesne, M.; Sichieri, R.; Bacaltchuk, J. "Double-Blind, Randomized, Placebo-Controlled Trial of Topiramate Plus Cognitive-Behavior Therapy in Binge-Eating Disorder." *Journal of Clinical Psychiatry*. (September 2007), 68 (9): 1324–1332.

Eichler, K.; Zoller, M.; Steurer, J.; Bachmann, L.M. "Cognitive-Behavioral Treatment for Weight Loss in Primary Care: A Prospective Study." *Swiss Medical Weekly*. (September 8, 2007), 137 (35–36): 489–495.

Munsch, S.; Biedert, E.; Meyer, A.; Michael, T.; Schlup, B.; Tuch, A.; Margraf, J. "A Randomized Comparison of Cognitive Behavioral Therapy and Behavioral Weight Loss Treatment for Overweight Individuals with Binge Eating Disorder." *International Journal of Eating Disorders*. (March 2007), 40 (2): 102–113.

Stahre, L.; Hallstrom, T. "A Short-Term Cognitive Group Treatment Program Gives Substantial Weight Reduction Up to 18 Months from the End of Treatment. A Randomized Controlled Trial." *Eating and Weight Disorders*. (March 2005), 10 (1): 51–58.

Stahre, L.; Tarnell, B.; Hakanson, C.E.; Hallstrom, T. "A Randomized Controlled Trial of Two Weight-Reducing Short-Term Group Treatment Programs for Obesity with an 18-Month Follow-Up." *International Journal of Behavioral Medicine*. (2007), 14 (1): 48–55.

Van den Akker, E.L.; Puiman, P.J.; Groen, M.; Timman, R.; Jongejan, M.T.; Trijsburg, W. "A Cognitive Behavioral Therapy Program for Overweight Children." *Journal of Pediatrics*. (September 2007), 151 (3): 280–283.

Wilson, G.T. "Psychological Treatment of Eating Disorders." *Annual Review of Clinical Psychology*. (2005), 1: 439–465.

## Chapter 2: Experience the Difference

Apolzan, J.; Carnell, N.; Mattes, R.; Campbell, W. "Inadequate Dietary Protein Increases Hunger and Desire to Eat in Younger and Older Men." *Journal of Nutrition*. (June 2007), 137 (6): 1478–1482.

Clifton, P.M.; Keogh, J.B.; Noakes, M. "Long-Term Effects of a High-Protein Weight-Loss Diet." *American Journal of Clinical Nutrition*. (January 2008), 87 (1): 23–29.

Clifton, P.M.; Noakes, M.; Keogh, J.; Foster, P. "Effect of an Energy Reduced High Protein Red Meat Diet on Weight Loss and Metabolic Parameters in Obese Women." *Asia Pacific Journal of Clinical Nutrition.* (2003), 12: S10.

Delzenne, N.M.; Cani, P.D. "A Place for Dietary Fiber in the Management of Metabolic Syndrome." *Current Opinion in Clinical Nutrition and Metabolic Care.* (November 2005), 8 (6): 636–640.

Howarth, N.C.; Saltzman, E.; Roberts, S.B. "Dietary Fiber and Weight Regulation." *Nutrition Reviews.* (May 2001), 59 (5): 129–139.

Leidy, H.J.; Carnell, N.S.; Mattes, R.D.; Campbell, W.W. "Higher Protein Intake Preserves Lean Mass and Satiety with Weight Loss in Pre-Obese and Obese Women." *Obesity (Silver Spring).* (February 2007), 5 (2): 421–429.

Noakes, M.; Keogh, J.B.; Foster, P.R.; Clifton, P.M. "Effect of an Energy-Restricted High-Protein, Low-Fat Diet Relative to a Conventional High-Carbohydrate, Low-Fat Diet on Weight Loss, Body Composition, Nutritional Status, and Markers of Cardiovascular Health in Obese Women." *American Journal of Clinical Nutrition.* (June 2005), 81 (6): 1298–1306.

Paniagua, J.A.; de la Sacristana, A.G.; Sánchez, E.; Romero, I.; Vidal-Puig, A.; Berral, F.J.; Escribano, A.; Moyano, M.J.; Peréz-Martinez, P.; López-Miranda, J.; Pérez-Jiménez, F. "A MUFA-Rich Diet Improves Posprandial Glucose, Lipid and GLP-1 Responses in Insulin-Resistant Subjects." *Journal of the American College of Nutrition.* (October 2007), 26 (5): 434–44.

Pereira, M.A.; Ludwig, D.S. "Dietary Fiber and Body Weight Regulation." *Pediatrics Clinics of North America.* (August 2001), 48 (4): 969–980.

Samra, R.A.; Anderson, G.H. "Insoluble Cereal Fiber Reduces Appetite and Short Term Food Intake and Glycemic Response to Food Consumed 75 Minutes Later by Healthy Men." *American Journal of Clinical Nutrition.* (October 2007), 86 (4): 972–979.

Vandewater, K.; Vickers, Z. "Higher-Protein Foods Produce Greater Sensory-Specific Satiety," *Physiology and Behavior.* (March 1996), 59 (3): 579–583.

## Chapter 3: Get Ready to Lose

Linde, J.A.; Jeffery, R.W.; Levy, R.L.; Pronk, N.P.; Boyle, R.G. "Weight Loss Goals and Treatment Outcomes Among Overweight Men and Women Enrolled in a Weight Loss Trial," *International Journal of Obesity.* (2005), 29: 1002–1005.

Orth, W.S.; Madan, A.K.; Taddeucci, R.J.; Coday, M.; Tichansky, D.S. "Support Group Meeting Attendance Is Associated with Better Weight Loss." *Obesity Surgery.* (April 2008), 18 (4): 391–394.

Svetkey, L.P.; Stevens, V.J.; Brantley, P.J.; Appel, L.J.; Hollis, J.F.; Loria, C.M.; Vollmer, W.M.; Gullion, C.M.; Funk, K.; Smith, P.; Samuel-Hodge, C.; Myers, V.; Lien, L.F.; Laferriere, D.; Kennedy, B.; Jerome, G.J.; Heinith, F.; Harsha, D.W.; Evans, P.; Erlinger, T.P.; Dalcin, A.T.; Coughlin, J.; Charleston, J.; Champagne, C.M.; Bauck, A.; Ard, J.D.; Aicher, K. Weight Loss Maintenance Collaborative Research Group. "Comparison of Strategies for Sustaining Weight Loss: The Weight Loss Maintenance Randomized Controlled Trial." *Journal of the American Medical Association.* (March 2008), 299 (10): 1139–1148.

Tate, D.F.; Jackvony, E.H.; Wing, R.R. "A Randomized Trial Comparing Human e-Mail Counseling, Computer-Automated Tailored Counseling, and No Counseling in an Internet Weight Loss Program." *Archives of Internal Medicine.* (2006), 166: 1620–1625.

Wansink, B.; Painter, J.E.; North, J. "Bottomless Bowls: Why Visual Cues of Portion Size May Influence Intake." *Obesity Research.* (January 2005), 13 (1): 93–100.

Wansink, B.; van Ittersum, K. "Bottoms Up! The Influence of Elongation on Pouring and Consumption Volume." *Journal of Consumer Research.* (December 2003), 30: 455–463.

Wansink, B.; van Ittersum, K. "Shape of Glass and Amount of Alcohol Poured: Comparative Study of Effect of Practice and Concentration." *British Medical Journal.* (January 2006), 331 (7531): 1512–1514.

## Chapter 4: Stage 1: The Success Skills Plan

Allison, A.; Melkus, G.; Chyun, D.; Galasso, P.; Wylie-Rossett, J. "Validation of Dietary Intake Data in Black Women with Type 2 Diabetes." *Journal of the American Dietetic Association.* (January 2007), 107 (1): 112–117.

Anderson, D.A.; Williamson, D.A.; Johnson, W.G.; Grieve, C.O. "Estimation of Food Intake: Effects of the Unit of Estimation." *Eating and Weight Disorders.* (March 1999), 4 (1): 6–9.

Bell, R.; Pliner, P.L. "Time to Eat: The Relationship Between the Number of People Eating and Meal Duration in Three Lunch Settings." *Appetite.* (October 2003), 41 (2): 215–218.

Brunstrom, J.M.; Mitchell, G.L. "Effects of Distraction on the Development of Satiety." *British Journal of Nutrition.* (October 2006), 96 (4): 761–769.

Cherkas, L.F.; Hunkin, J.L.; Kato, B.S.; Richards, J.B.; Gardner, J.P.; Surdulescu, G.L.; Kimura, M.; Lu, X.; Spector, T.D.; Aviv, A. "The Association Between Physical Activity in Leisure Time and Leukocyte Telomere Length." *Archives of Internal Medicine.* (January 2008), 168 (2): 154–158.

Cousins, S.O. "A Self Referent Thinking Model: How Older Adults May Talk Themselves Out of Being Physically Active." *Health Promotion Practice.* (October 2003), 4 (4): 439–448.

Farshchi, H.R.; Taylor, M.A.; Macdonald, I.A. "Beneficial Metabolic Effects of Regular Meal Frequency on Dietary Thermogenesis, Insulin Sensitivity, and Fasting Lipid Profiles in Healthy, Obese Women." *American Journal of Clinical Nutrition.* (January 2005), 81 (1): 16–24.

Farshchi, H.R.; Taylor, M.A.; Macdonald, I.A. "Decreased Thermic Effect of Food After an Irregular Compared to a Regular Meal Pattern in Healthy Lean Women." *International Journal of Obesity Related Medical Disorders.* (May 2004), 28 (5): 653–660.

Hoffman, M.D.; Hoffman, D.R. "Exercisers Achieve Greater Acute Exercise-Induced Mood Enhancement Than Nonexercisers." *Archives of Physical Medicine and Rehabilitation.* (February 2008), 89 (2): 358–363.

Kaplan, D.L. "Eating Style of Obese and Nonobese Males." *Psychosomatic Medicine.* (November 1980), 42 (6): 529–538.

Klem, M.L.; Wing, R.R.; McGuire, M.T.; Seagle, H.M.; Hill, J.O. "A Descriptive Study of Individuals Successful at Long-Term Maintenance of Substantial Weight Loss." *American Journal of Clinical Nutrition.* (August 1997), 66 (2): 239–246.

Linde, J.A.; Jeffery, R.W.; French, S.A.; Pronk, N.P.; Boyle, R.G. "Self-Weighing in Weight Gain Prevention and Weight Loss Trials." *Annals of Behavioral Medicine.* (2005), 30 (3): 210–216.

Martins, C.; Robertson, M.D.; Morgan, L.M. "Effects of Exercise and Restrained Eating Behaviour on Appetite Control." *The Proceedings of the Nutrition Society.* (February 2008), 67 (1): 28–41.

McFarlane, T.; Polivy, J.; Peter, H.C. "Effects of False Weight Feedback on Mood, Self Evaluation, and Food Intake in Restrained and Unrestrained Eaters." *Journal of Abnormal Psychology.* (May 1998), 107 (2): 312–318.

Pinto, A.M.; Heinberg, L.J.; Coughlin, J.W.; Fava, J.L.; Guarda, A.S. "The Eating Disorder Recovery Self-Efficacy Questionnaire (EDRSQ): Change with Treatment and Prediction of Outcome." *Eating Behaviors.* (April 2008), 9 (2): 143–153.

Pliner, P.; Zec, D. "Meal Schemas During a Preload Decrease Subsequent Eating." *Appetite.* (May 2007), 48 (3): 278–288.

Puetz, T.W.; Flowers, S.S.; O'Connor, P.J. "A Randomized Controlled Trial of the Effect of Aerobic Exercise Training on Feelings of Energy and Fatigue in Sedentary Young Adults with Persistent Fatigue." *Psychotherapy and Psychosomatics.* (February 2008), 77 (3): 167–174.

Raynor, D.A.; Phelan, S.; Hill, J.O.; Wing, R. "Television Viewing and Long-Term Weight Maintenance: Results from the National Weight Control Registry." *Obesity.* (October 2006), 14 (10): 1816–1824.

Schoeller, D.A. "Limitations in the Assessment of Dietary Energy Intake by Self Report." *Metabolism: Clinical & Experimental.* (1995), 44 (2 Suppl 2): 18–22.

Smith, B.W.; Shelley, B.M.; Leahigh, L.; Vanleit, B. "A Preliminary Study of the Effects of a Modified Mindfulness Intervention on Binge Eating." *Complementary Health Practice Review.* (October 2006), 11 (3): 133–143.

Speechly, D.P.; Rogers, G.G.; Buffenstein, R. "Acute Appetite Reduction Associated with an Increased Frequency of Eating in Obese Males." *International Journal of Obesity Related Metabolic Disorders.* (November 1999), 23 (11): 1151–1159.

Wansink, B. "Environmental Factors That Increase the Food Intake and Consumption Volume of Unknowing Consumers." *Annual Reviews in Nutrition.* (2004), 24: 455–479.

Wing, R.R.; Tate, D.F.; Gorin, A.A.; Raynor, H.A.; Fava, J.L.; Machan, J. "STOP Regain: Are There Negative Effects of Daily Weighing?" *Journal of Consulting and Clinical Psychology.* (August 2007), 75 (4): 652–656.

Wooley, O.W.; Wooley, S.C.; Turner, K. "The Effects of Rate of Consumption on Appetite in the Obese and Nonobese." *Recent Advances in Obesity Research.* (1975), 1: 212–215.

## Chapter 5: Stage 2: The Think Thin Initial Eating Plan

Bravata, D.M.; Smith-Spangler, C.; Sundaram, V. "Using Pedometers to Increase Physical Activity and Health: A Systematic Review." *Journal of the American Medical Association.* (November 2007), 298 (19): 2296–2304.

Farshchi, H.R.; Taylor, M.A.; Macdonald, I.A. "Deleterious Effects of Omitting Breakfast on Insulin Sensitivity and Fasting Lipid Profiles in Healthy, Lean Women." *American Journal of Clinical Nutrition.* (February 2005), 81 (2): 388–396.

Harnack, L.; Steffen, L.; Arnett, D.; Gao, S.; Luepker, R. "Accuracy of Estimation of Large Food Portions." *Journal of the American Dietetic Association.* (May 2004), 104 (5): 804–806.

Klem, M.L.; Wing, R.R.; McGuire, M.T.; Seagle, H.M.; Hill, J.O. "A Descriptive Study of Individuals Successful at Long-Term Maintenance of Substantial Weight Loss." *American Journal of Clinical Nutrition.* (August 1997), 66 (2): 239–246.

Klesges, R.; Eck, L.; Ray, J. "Who Underreports Dietary Intake in a Dietary Recall? Evidence from the Second National Health and Nutrition Examination Survey." *Journal of Consulting and Clinical Psychology.* (June 1995), 63 (3): 438–444.

Levitsky, D.A. "The Non-Regulation of Food Intake in Humans: Hope for Reversing the Epidemic of Obesity." *Physiology & Behavior.* (2005), 86: 623–632.

Miller, D.L.; Bell, E.A.; Pelkman, C.L,; Peters, J.C.; Rolls, B.J. "Effects of Dietary Fat, Nutrition Labels, and Repeated Consumption on Sensory-Specific Satiety." *Physiology & Behavior.* (October 15, 2000), 71 (1–2): 153–158.

Purslow, L.R.; Sandhu, M.S.; Forouhi, N.; Young, E.H.; Luben, R.N.; Welch, A.A.; Khaw, K.T.; Bingham, S.A.; Wareham, N.J. "Energy Intake at Breakfast and Weight Change: Prospective Study of 6,764 Middle-Aged Men and Women." *American Journal of Epidemiology.* (January 15, 2008), 167 (2): 188–192.

Raynor, H.A.; Epstein, L.H. "Dietary Variety, Energy Regulation and Obesity." *Psychological Bulletin.* (May 2001), 127 (3): 325–341.

Raynor, H.A.; Jeffery, R.W.; Phelan, S.; Hill, J.O.; Wing, R.R. "Amount of Food Group Variety Consumed in the Diet and Long-Term Weight Loss Maintenance." *Obesity Research.* (May 2005), 13 (5): 883–890.

Raynor, H.A.; Niemeier, H.M.; Wing, R.R. "Effect of Limiting Snack Food Variety on Long-Term Sensory-Specific Satiety and Monotony During Obesity Treatment." *Eating Behaviors.* (January 2006), 7 (1): 1–14.

Raynor, H.A.; Wing, R.R. "Effect of Limiting Snack Food Variety Across Days on Hedonics and Consumption." *Appetite.* (March 2006), 46 (2): 168–176.

Rolls, B.J.; Bell, E.A.; Thorwart, M.L. "Water Incorporated into a Food but Not Served with a Food Decreases Energy Intake in Lean Women." *American Journal of Clinical Nutrition.* (October 1999), 70 (4): 448–455.

Rolls, B.J.; Roe, L.S.; Meengs, J.S. "Salad and Satiety: Energy Density and Portion Size of a First-Course Salad Affect Energy Intake at Lunch." *Journal of the American Dietetic Association.* (October 2004), 104 (10): 1570–1576.

Van der Heijden, A.A.; Hu, F.B.; Rimm, E.B.; van Dam, R.M. "A Prospective Study of Breakfast Consumption and Weight Gain Among U.S. Men." *Obesity.* (October 2007), 15 (10): 2463–2469.

Vandewater, K.; Vickers, Z. "Higher-Protein Foods Produce Greater Sensory-Specific Satiety." *Physiology & Behavior.* (March 1996), 59 (3): 579–583.

Wansink, B. "Environmental Factors That Increase the Food Intake and Consumption Volume of Unknowing Consumers." *Annual Reviews in Nutrition.* (2004), 24: 455–479.

Wansink, B.; Chandon, P. "Meal Size, Not Body Size, Explains Errors in Estimating the Calorie Content of Meals." *Annals of Internal Medicine.* (September 2006), 145 (5): 326–332.

Wansink, B.; Cheney, M.M.; Chan, N. "Exploring Comfort Food Preferences Across Age and Gender." *Physiology & Behavior.* (2003), 79: 739–747.

Wansink, B.; van Ittersum, K.; Painter, J. "Ice Cream Illusions: Bowls, Spoons and Self-Served Portion Sizes." *American Journal of Preventive Medicine.* (September 2006), 31 (4): 240–243.

Wyatt, H.R.; Grunwald, G.K.; Mosca, C.L.; Klem, M.L.; Wing, R.R.; Hill, J.O. "Long-Term Weight Loss and Breakfast in Subjects in the National Weight Control Registry." *Obesity Research.* 10: 78–82.

## Chapter 6: Stage 3: The Challenging Situations Plan

Binkley, J.K.; Eales, J.; Jekanowski, M. "The Relation Between Dietary Change and Rising U.S. Obesity." *International Journal of Obesity.* (August 2000), 24 (8): 1032–1039.

Duerksen, S.C.; Elder, J.P.; Arredondo, E.M.; Ayala, G.X.; Slyman, D.J.; Campbell, N.R.; Baquero, B. "Family Restaurant Choices are Associated with Child and Adult Overweight Status in Mexican-American Families." *Journal of the American Dietetic Association.* (May 2007), 107 (5): 849–853.

Gorin, A.A.; Phelan, S.; Wing, R.R.; Hill, H.O. "Promoting Long-Term Weight Control: Does Dieting Consistency Matter?" *International Journal of Obesity.* (2004), 28 (2): 278–281.

Harnack, L.; Steffen, L.; Arnett, D.; Gao, S.; Luepker, R. "Accuracy of Estimation of Large Food Portions." *Journal of the American Dietetic Association.* (May 2004), 104 (5): 804–806.

Kant, A.K.; Graubard, B.I. "Eating Out in America 1987–2000: Trends and Nutritional Correlates." *Preventive Medicine.* (February 2004), 38 (2): 243–249.

Mehta, N.K.; Chang, V.W. "Weight Status and Restaurant Availability: A Multilevel Analysis." *American Journal of Preventive Medicine.* (February 1998), 34 (2): 127–133.

Wansink, B. "Environmental Factors That Increase the Food Intake and Consumption Volume of Unknowing Consumers." *Annual Reviews in Nutrition.* (2004), 24: 455–479.

## Chapter 8: Stage 5: The Motivation-for-Life Plan

Klem, M.L.; Wing, R.R.; Lang, W.; McGuire, M.T.; Hill, J.O. "Does Weight Loss Maintenance Become Easier Over Time?" *Obesity Research.* (2000), 8: 438–444.

Phelan, S.; Hill, J.O.; Lang, W.; Dibello, J.; Wing, R.R. "Recovery from Relapse Among Successful Weight Maintainers." *The American Journal of Clinical Nutrition.* (December 2003), 78 (6): 1079–1084.

Phelan, S.; Wyatt, H.R.; Hill, J.O.; Wing, R.R. "Are the Eating and Exercise Habits of Successful Weight Losers Changing?" *Obesity.* (April 2006), 14 (4): 710–716.

# Index